Advances in Anatomy Embryology and Cell Biology

Vol. 171

Springer

Berlin
Heidelberg
New York
Hong Kong
London
Milan
Paris
Tokyo

Restoring Function
to the Injured Human Spinal Cord

Richard Ben Borgens
Mari Hulman George Professor of Applied Neurology,
School of Veterinary Medicine
Professor of Biomedical Engineering,
School of Engineering
Purdue University,
West Lafayette, Indiana 47907, USA
(765) 494-7600
Fax: (765) 494-7605
e-mail: cpr@purdue.edu

Illustrator:
Kimberly J. Harrington
Center for Paralysis Research,
Department of Basic Medical Sciences
School of Veterinary Medicine
Purdue University,
West Lafayette, Indiana 47907, USA

I dedicate this Book to the Memory
of Melvin Cohen
Professor of Biology
Yale University
Professor Cohen taught me to dream with optimism
about the potential for the New Biology
to change the quality of lives of paralyzed people
But through hard work and careful experimentation
He will be greatly missed

Acknowledgements

This text describes many experiments and clinical trials, none of which would be possible without the dedication and *esprit de corps* of so many people along the way: My colleague of 16 years, Debra Bohnert; and my scientific/faculty colleagues Ernesto Roederer, Riyi Shi, Andrew Blight, James Toombs, Rick Widmer, Gert Breur, Chandra Bajaj, John Turek, and Kimbal Pratt. As an apprentice scientist, one owes much to their mentors – I had the best: David Redden, Lionel Jaffe, Melvin Cohen, and Richmond Prehn. Some of my students and colleagues contributed so much to these investigations, as well as the energy, scholarship, and creativity behind them: Mary Elizabeth Metcalf, Riyi Shi, Bradley Duerstock, Loren Moriarty, Alicia Altizer, Jill Donaldson, and Alenka Leskovar.

The clinical trials in canine paraplegia would not have been possible without the dedicated spirit of the staff of the Purdue University Department of Veterinary Clinical Sciences, and the Student Hospital – and more recently, a similar group of technicians, faculty, and surgical residents at Texas A&M University, School of Veterinary Medicine. Not to be forgotten are those owners of paraplegic dogs that entered into these veterinary clinical trials, cared for their animals, and ultimately, made these experiments a success.

The human clinical trials would not have been possible without old friends Robert Hansebout, McMaster University School of Medicine and Keith Hayes at the University of Western Ontario School of Medicine – and new friends Scott Shapiro, Paul Nelson, and Robert Pascuzzi at the Indiana University School of Medicine. These neurosurgeons and neurologists took our ideas, made them safe and practical for the human patient, and applied them as experimental tools.

The oil and gas of the scientific machine in this modern era is funding. I acknowledge the generous and long time support of this research by the Public Health Service, National Institutes of Health and The Center for Injury Control, The Department of Defense, and the National Science Foundation. We owe much to sustaining support of our Institute by the State of Indiana, the Office of the Governor, Frank O'Bannon, Representative William Cochran, State Senator Morris Mills, and Representative Cleo Duncan, and to the volunteer organization for support of those persons in need in the State of Indiana, COVOH, and especially its Chairwoman, Ms. Amy Cook Lurvey. Generous financial support from the Spinal Cord Society, President Charles Carson and Vice President Dick Stonestrom gave our spinal cord research center its start in 1987. Intel Corporation has long been generous to our research group through donations of computer hardware.

I humbly acknowledge the great personal generosities of Mrs. Helen Skinner, and Ms. Mari Hulman George through their financial endowments to this University in support of our research.

Finally, two people did the real work of organizing and preparing this manuscript for publication: Ms. Carie Brackenbury, and Ms. Charlyce Patterson.

Contents

Foreword

This book has two major themes: one, to provide a general understanding of the biology of spinal cord injury (SCI) in animal models and their relationship to naturally occurring injury in man, and secondly, to review novel means to induce functional recovery from spinal cord injury based on developmental biophysics and physiology. These are new innovations in the treatment of SCI, born of disciplines that have not received much attention from investigators interested in the repair and regeneration of the Central Nervous System (CNS). They include development of 4-Aminopyridine for chronic SCI; oscillating electrical fields and polymer infusion for acute SCI. Biochemistry, neurotransplantation techniques, and pharmacological approaches have long dominated this literature. Curiously though, it is these former techniques that are more practical and are rapidly moving into human clinical studies, or have already begun then. All of these clinical therapies have been developed at the Center for Paralysis Research at Purdue University, mirroring the backgrounds and interests of the electrophysiologists and biophysicists of our Research Center's faculty. Two of the three experimental therapies for SCI developed at Purdue University are now in human clinical trials, and a third will soon begin. They frame the emphasis of this text.

To properly evaluate these studies, sufficient background covering the history and biology of spinal cord injury, a discussion of the limits to our presumptions concerning realistic clinical therapies derived from animal models of SCI, and an introductory primer on the human injury need to be provided for the interested reader. This is a rather ambitious undertaking – one that could easily lead to a much larger book – and one not easily appreciated by scientists and students from many different backgrounds. Thus, I have constructed this monograph differently than the typical scholarly review.

First, for those who expect many hundreds of citations, even multiple ones referencing every declarative statement, they will find this bibliography perhaps scant compared to the size of the text. Important or controversial subject matter will, of course, be cited in this text. More common and/or well-accepted issues will not. Many times I have not used the most recent citation(s) to reference work or ideas, choosing instead to use either the seminal papers behind certain observations, or reports that I believe to be the most informative. A few helpful reviews will be cited – even if they are not the most recent. I have found that exhaustive citations sometimes spoil the narrative, and I am not fond of reviews citing other reviews.

In the last decade or two, (scholarly) reviews have become simply summaries or lists of the subject matter. It is no longer (politically) correct to critically evaluate the results of experiments, or to offer an opinion if they pass muster. In this text, the most influential subjects will receive such a close look – but others may not, receiving something of a free pass. This reflects my subjective opinion of what is important. One of the great strengths of writing a monograph is that one does not have to placate the opinions of other co-authors – however, I freely admit this is also one of its weaknesses. Overall, this style reflects my individual biases after more than 32 years of reading and writing about science.

I have tried to use as little jargon as possible in this text, and explain some of the more fundamental issues in biology and medicine so that *all* readers may appreciate this exciting area of research. Spinal cord injury is a complicated pathology requiring an appreciation of studies from the molecular level to the behavior of the whole animal. Thus, for example, the gross anatomy is presented in a simplified fashion for the cell and molecular biologist, while I have tried to do the reverse for the anatomist or surgeon. I understand this will be to light of a touch for some readers, but perhaps heavy going for others. I have tried to strike a balance between these.

Each figure is a lesson unto itself. Each figure is important to understanding the narrative, and should not to be considered as simply documentation of statements made in the text. The figures are constructed with some artistic license and sometimes large legends – because they each tell a story. They also provide explanation about issues that, when included in the body of the text, produce too much of a digression. Finally, I hope this monograph is fundamentally useful to many persons – not just those "skilled in the art". This is a goal guiding its construction. Indeed, modern neurobiology is now turning the corner on a 50 year history of failed treatments designed to improve the quality of life for those surviving SCI – and I hope this story will be both a timely one, and an interesting one, for all.

1 A Brief Primer on Spinal Cord Injury

Injuries to the central nervous system (CNS), the brain and spinal cord, are arguably the worst survivable injuries to the human body. Prior to World War II, such injuries were death sentences. Spinal cord injuries were hardly treated surgically in the First World War; injured persons were left to die. During the Second World War, a more enlightened approach was pursued, and the early beginnings of special spinal cord injury (SCI) management and rehabilitation began (Bedbrook 1987). The availability of modern antibiotics after the war and progressive improvement in clinical management lengthened the lives of injured people, but did not improve their outcome. This area of research, in my opinion, is the last frontier for the medicine of trauma. A decade ago, substantial third-degree burns could be a death sentence. Now there are artificial skins replating denuded regions of the body and saving lives. Over a decade ago, a chronic fracture nonunion that continually failed to respond to management would lead to amputation. Today this is rarely the outcome. There has been no such movement in the area of CNS trauma management. Even the much ballyhooed administration of high dosages of a steroid – methylprednisolone sodium succinate (Bracken et al. 1990) – has fallen on hard times and may not survive as a treatment of choice (discussed in Chap. 4, "Treating the Acute and Chronic Injury: Historical Perspective"; see Short et al. 2000; Pointillant et al. 2000).

In the 1950s, the conventional management of SCI was to surgically decompress the region of the injury, removing any offending material (bone chips, prolapsed disc material, etc.) and to stabilize the vertebral column, if required, through the use of orthopedic fixation techniques and spine fusion. This is still the standard of care for spinal injured people. While there have indeed been improvements in fixation devices, surgical techniques, and rehabilitation techniques (Theodore and Sonntag 2000), a novel biological approach to the medical treatment of paralyzed people – proven to substantially improve their neurological outcome – has not been discovered.

1.1
Epidemiology

The most thorough evaluation of SCI occurred in the mid 1990s and has been amended only slightly since then (DeVivo et al. 1995; Berkowitz et al. 1998). Estimates of the numbers of chronically injured persons are on the order of 250,000–350,000. SCI occurs in at least 10,000–12,000 persons annually in the United States. The average age at injury is approximately 31, while the most frequently occurring age at injury (the mode) is 19 years. Roughly 80% of the injured are male (Go et al. 1995). Spinal cord and head injury is epidemic amongst young adults. It is born of vehicular accidents and general risk taking in sports and outdoor activities. This catastrophic change in life occurs before most injured people have finished their education, before they have severed ties with home, before they have achieved independent living, before they have settled into stable employment, or achieved significant medical benefits. The injury plunges them into a life of dependence and sometimes poverty. It may bankrupt their families. Spinal cord injury breaks not only bodies – but also families, marriages, and dreams.

An insidious demographic trend has also emerged at the end of the twentieth century, worsening this bleak picture. In urban areas, acts of violence increasingly contribute to CNS injury. In some socioeconomic groups, the epidemiological data are already alarmingly skewed. For example, gunshot wounds to young black men 20 years and younger have surpassed vehicular accidents as the leading cause of SCI in some samples. Such high velocity, penetrating injuries to the spinal cord are the least tractable of all injuries. First-year direct medical costs for SCI have spiraled upwards – and continue to do so – approaching $500,000 per case. However, in the ever-increasing SCIs related to violence, where numerous other organ systems are injured (usually by gunshot), initial hospitalization and rehabilitation costs can approach and exceed $1 million. In a cover story entitled "Killer Costs" appearing in *US News and World Report* (April 1998), several such SCI cases were profiled, ranging from $500,000 to $1,200,000 for initial bills. The point was made that the costs of these crime-related injuries are passed on nearly completely to state and federal governments. Though I am an avid collector of historical firearms, I have to admit that better and tighter control of handguns in the United States would more cheaply and rapidly reduce the incidence of SCI, the suffering, and the societal costs of this injury than medical research.

Even though SCI is less frequent than other types of injury and disease, the costs to individuals and society are unexpectedly staggering. This is due in part to the low age at injury coupled with the increasing life expectancies of those injured. The most recent studies suggest indirect costs (lost wages, productivity, fringe benefits, etc.) plus direct costs produce an aggregate cost to society between $7 and $10 billion annually (Berkowitz 1998; DeVivo et al. 1995). At present there are no known treatments that can alter the biology of this injury to significantly change the axis of behavioral deficits produced by it. In spite of other advancements (Bracken et al. 1990; Geisler et al.1991), we should view the opportunity for significant improvement in the behavioral loss following severe CNS neurotrauma as limited and the quality of life for those affected as impoverished.

To the general public, severe brain injury is relatively easy to understand as a catastrophe given the injured person's intellectual and cognitive impairments in addition to the physical disability. Sometimes SCI is more difficult for the layman to evaluate. It was once commonly perceived that persons with spinal injuries were relatively normal, they just could not walk. This skewed view of paraplegia (actually ~70% of SCI results in quadriplegia) was strengthened by television commercials of the 1980s and 1990s featuring healthy looking paraplegics playing wheelchair sports and guzzling cola wearing prominent athletic wrist bands. The injury to the actor Christopher Reeve has at least brought the true horror of SCI into focus in the national consciousness.

2 The Behavioral Catastrophe Is Rooted in Injury to White Matter

2.1
The Ground Plan of the Spinal Cord

The biological basis for the functional loss accompanying spinal cord injury is mostly rooted in the loss of nerve impulse conduction (electrical traffic) through the lesion in injured white matter (Blight 1991; Folis et al. 1993). White matter owes its name to its staining characteristics as studied by the nineteenth century anatomist. This light staining was due to high concentrations of myelin, a fatty substance insulating most spinal cord nerve fibers or axons. White matter is comprised of myelinated and unmyelinated axons, many organized into numerous tracts, collective bundles of nerve processes coursing in the same direction to common target regions of the nervous system. This region is comprised solely of the processes of nerve cells (and not their cell bodies) surrounding the centrally located gray matter (darker in staining due to the presence of the nerve cell bodies). The connection between brain and body is made possible by the direction of nerve impulse traffic in the so-called long-tract pathways of white matter. Sensory information projects into the spinal cord via sensory nerve fibers that ascend the spinal cord to the base of the brain, while motor nerve impulse traffic (for example, initiating volitional movement) leaves the brain by descending the spinal cord in organized tracts of nerve fibers in the white matter.

Many of the localized bundles or tracts of nerve fibers spanning the spinal cord are associated with characteristic functions that have been identified by scientists for over 100 years. For example, the sensory appreciation of vibration and light touch applied to the skin ascends the spinal cord in bilaterally organized long tracts, the dorsal column pathway. Another ascending tract, the spinothalamic tract, carries the sense of temperature and pain. These tracts are localized to different parts of the spinal cord, and take different pathways as they ascend the cord. They pass through identified regions within the brain to their final destination – the sensory cortex – making numerous synapses with second- and third-order neurons that are part of this chain along the way.

Descending motor control can also be restricted to organized long tracts such as the control of muscular activity of the extremities carried by the corticospinal tract (Fig. 1). The anatomical organization associated with other functions may be more diffuse, even unidentified. Examples of functions carried by such diffuse nerve projections within the cord include the sensation of deep pain that originates in special-

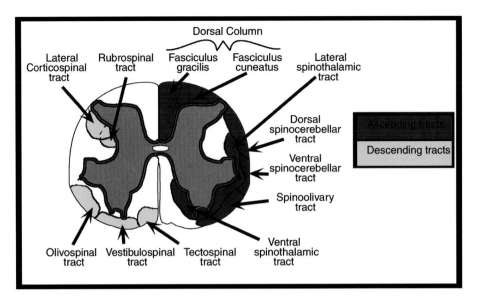

Fig. 1. Anatomy of the human spinal cord; ascending and descending tracts. Note the familiar appearance of the gray matter in cross section. The location of a few of the major ascending and descending tracts in the surrounding white matter are shown. These bilateral long tract columns of nerve fibers traverse much of the length of the cord. The two components of the dorsal column are shown, the fasciculus cuneatus and gracilis. The former builds its substance upon the entry of sensory nerves from the extremities at each dorsal root as axons are added laterally with each ascending vertebral level. Both of these tracts terminate in the hindbrain at the nucleus cuneatus and gracilis. They convey the sense of light touch and vibration, among other sensations. Another ascending sensory tract discussed in the text, the spinothalamic, is also found in two components bilaterally ascending the spinal cord. It conveys the senses of superficial pain and temperature, among others sensations. Descending tracts originate from first order neurons in the brain. Descending tracts discussed in the text include the vestibulospinal tract, involving balance and posture, and the corticospinal tract, projecting to motor neurons in the cord. It is the interruption in nerve impulse traffic traveling in these ascending and descending pathways that results in the catastrophic behavioral loss associated with spinal cord injury

Fig. 2A,B. The spine and spinal cord of humans. A The man at the *top right* shows the relative position of the bony vertebral column or spine and its four basic divisions (named to the *right* of the silhouette). Note the normal curvature of the spine with convex (lordosis) and concave (kyphosis) portions. The vertebral column contains the spinal cord, which is shown in the exploded view in **B**. The vertebral segments of each of the four subdivisions (cervical through sacral) are both *color-coded* and *numbered* in the key to the *right* of the spine. Of the five sacral vertebrae, the last three segments are fused. Note that the spinal cord of humans ends at L1. Spinal roots at lower levels project downward through, and out of, the remaining vertebrae as the cauda equina, or horse's tail

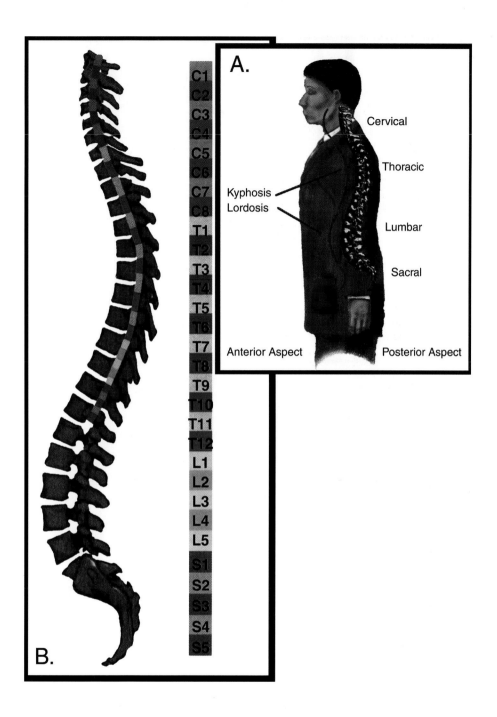

A.

Cervical

Thoracic

Kyphosis
Lordosis

Lumbar

Sacral

Anterior Aspect

Posterior Aspect

B.

C1
C2
C3
C4
C5
C6
C7
C8
T1
T2
T3
T4
T5
T6
T7
T8
T9
T10
T11
T12
L1
L2
L3
L4
L5
S1
S2
S3
S4
S5

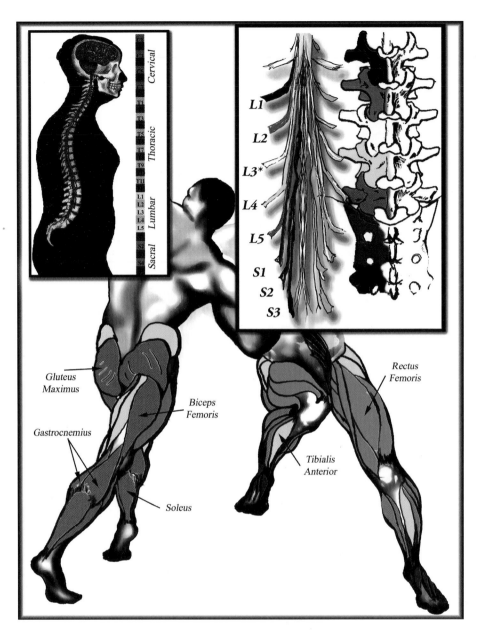

Fig. 3. The spinal cord, levels of injury, and paraplegia. The *inset* to the *left* repeats some of the anatomy shown in Fig. 2; however, the two components of the CNS, the brain and spinal cord, are *highlighted*. Note again, in the *inset* to the *right*, that the human spinal cord ends at L1. The spinal nerves at this level and below continue to project downwards towards the tip of the sacrum, exiting at the vertebral segments shown. These are *color-coded* for the sacral levels where the ventral spinal roots exit the vertebral column (for simplicity, only the left side is rendered). The major muscles of the lower extremities that receive these bilateral motor nerve fibers from L1 to S3 are *color-coded* to the vertebral levels servicing them. These muscles, especially the larger ones, receive motor neuron

ized sensory receptors of muscle and tendon, or the descending nerve projections associated with inhibition of motor nerves within the spinal cord gray matter.

The nerve fibers projecting out to the muscles of the extremities take their origin from neurons located in intumescences (or swollen regions) of the spinal cord, roughly equivalent to the upper extremities (the cervical enlargement, C4 to T2) or the lower extremities (the lumbar intumescence, a.k.a. the lumbosacral enlargement; L1 to S2; refer to Fig. 2). Motor neurons located in these intumescences are the source of axons coursing out to musculature via the trunks of peripheral nerves. These nerve trunks, when proximal to the vertebral column, are the segmentally organized spinal roots. Recall that for every muscle, particularly large ones of the extremities, the individual motor units of muscle are innervated by the axons arising from motor neurons in several contiguous (up to four) vertebral segments (Fig. 3). Thus, loss of motor neurons innervating a muscle originating from only one vertebral segment (most clinical injuries to the spinal cord are less than one vertebral segment in extent) is associated with muscle weakness (paresis) and not paralysis.

In fact, localized, rather complete destruction of gray matter occurs in the clinical condition central cord syndrome (Tator 1995). This is not characteristic of paraplegia or quadriplegia but paresis (a weakening of limbs). For this and other reasons, I emphasize, both here and throughout this monograph, that spinal cord injury resulting in quadriplegia or paraplegia is a white matter injury. It is the interruption of the long tract communication system between body and brain that segments or compartmentalizes the injured body into two regions: functional and nonfunctional. When this disconnection occurs in the cervical area (that is, above the level of cervical enlargement; refer also to Fig. 2), quadriplegia results. When this injury occurs below the intumescences in the upper thoracic to lumbar region, paraplegia is the result. In a "neurologically complete" injury, all voluntary motor control below the level of the injury is lost, as is all normally experienced sensation arising from below the lesion. Behaviorally, it is as if the spinal cord was cut into two pieces, so complete may be the compartmentalization – or segmentation – of the body. This is probably why many neurosurgeons may tell patients and their families the cord is severed, because this is how it may appear to them. However, usually the cord is not anatomically transected, a very rare occurrence.

---

input from two to four continuous vertebral levels. Only the first of these is *color-coded*, and only a few of the larger muscles are named for simplicity. The *asterisk* at L3 notes that motor neurons first projecting from this level connect with deep muscles of the legs (not shown in the drawing). This drawing reveals that with each ascending level of injury, more and more portions of the muscles of the legs are compromised by injury to the spinal cord. With complete injuries above L1, most of the limb musculature would be completely paralyzed. This is because all of the nerves shown, projecting out of the spine to the musculature of the legs, become isolated from the descending motor projections from higher levels of the cord and the brain. This results in paraplegia. Injuries in the cervical region above the cervical intumescence (cervical enlargement, not shown) isolates motor projections to the arms, as well as the legs, resulting in quadriplegia (sometimes referred to as tetraplegia)

2.2
Characteristics of Spinal Cord Injury

The initial cause of the damage to spinal cord tissue (a.k.a. parenchyma) is biomechanical. Forces are directed onto the cord, usually through acute compression (Yoganandan et al. 1999; Tuszynski et al. 1999; Fig. 4). In fact, the typical spinal cord injury results in a rind of spared spinal cord tissue of variable thickness, though this anatomically intact parenchyma is physiologically nonfunctional in the most severe cases. We will follow up this observation in subsequent sections since spared but nonfunctional white matter provides an interesting and overlooked therapeutic avenue.

Neurologically incomplete individuals exhibit some residual motor and/or sensory preservation after the injury, likely associated with functional white matter surviving the insult. This can be detected by the neurologist after allowing a variable time for spinal shock to subside. This latter term applies to the reversible loss of spinal reflexes following the acute event. No matter how minor this sparing of function may be, however, it indicates a better functional outcome for the patient in response to rehabilitation than will occur in neurologically complete cases.

Spinal injury also leads to loss or imbalance in numerous involuntary functions such as defecation and voiding reflexes, breathing, and even the control of blood pressure, depending on the vertebral level where the injury was sustained (Ditunno and Formal 1994). Generally speaking, the higher (or closer to the head) the spinal injury– the more remarkable the behavioral loss (Figs. 2, 3). Even life-threatening conditions can arise from the compartmentalization of involuntary functioning of the autonomic nervous system after the injury. For example, the vagal (parasympathetic) control of heart activity in humans may remain intact with lesions to the cord (the vagus nerve projects to the body from the upper neck in close association with the foramen of the jugular vein and internal carotid artery). However, the sympathetic control of the heart arises from sympathetic neurons of the thoracic gray matter of the spinal cord. Thus, an injury between the two anatomically separates the involuntary circuits that normally work in concert with each other to balance heart activity. Autonomic dysreflexia, sometimes manifested as an uncontrolled and dangerous spiking of blood pressure, arises from unopposed sympathetic stimulation (Fig. 5).

Bowel and bladder functioning is also based on reflex activity, localized to reflex circuits in the sacral spinal cord. These reflexes are modified, however, by descending (supraspinal) inhibition from the brain, which provides voluntary control of voiding and evacuation. This control is disconnected after spinal injury, resulting in incontinence. Furthermore, respiratory function is not just accomplished by the action of the diaphragm, but by accessory musculature as well. This includes the intercostal muscles of the ribs and abdominal musculature (Fig. 6). Even if the innervation of the diaphragm survives spinal injury intact, higher-level injuries still severely compromise breathing because control of this accessory musculature is lost, as discussed in the legend to Fig. 6.

Usually the damage to spinal cord is produced by mechanical force, sometimes accompanying damage to the cord's parenchyma by bony fragments and disc material, and usually always accompanied by localized hemorrhage (Fig. 4). As mentioned, human pathological studies reveal that this is usually a localized lesion and restricted

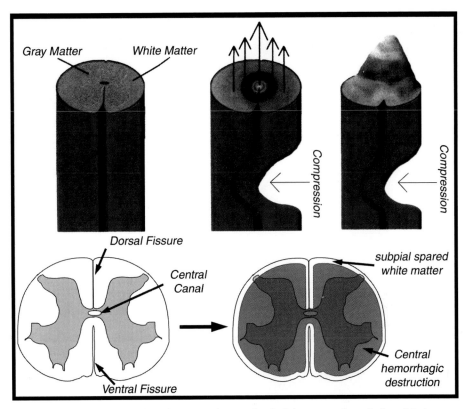

Fig. 4. Spinal cord and spinal cord compression. Mechanical damage to the spinal cord in humans usually arises from compression, not transection. The tissue of the spinal cord may be lacerated by bony fragments arising from the shattered vertebral column (as in burst fractures of the spine), or hyperextended or stretched (as in neck injuries); however, the most prevalent force causing spinal paralysis in humans is due to a deformation of the spine and the resulting compression of the cord within it. This produces a focus of tissue damage that, in some sense, is counterintuitive. Instead of the cord being mostly damaged at its surface (where the impact is first experienced), it is most severely damaged in central regions. This injury to the tissue continues to expand outward, or centrifugal, with time. In a phrase, the spinal cord is injured "inside-out." This is illustrated by the physical principle that compression of a cylinder (the spinal cord) containing a soft or liquid substance (the tissues of the cord) produces the most distortion of that substance in the center of the cylinder along its long axis. Thus, gray matter within the surrounding white matter of the spinal cord can be largely destroyed. A variable rim, or rind, of white matter closest to the surface of the spinal cord is usually spared. This is illustrated in the cross sections, beginning with a normal cord before compression and after. The forces exerted on the center produces hemorrhage, and since the gray matter is more vascularized than white matter, it is most vulnerable. For illustrative purposes, the cross-sectional views at the *bottom* do not show the distortion of the cord due to compression, and the amount and location of white matter sparing is extremely variable from one cord to the next after injury

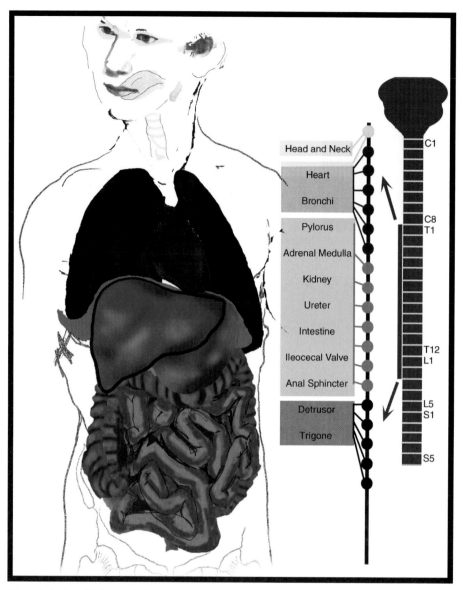

Fig. 5. Spinal cord injury and the autonomic control of the organs and viscera. The involuntary control of organs by the autonomic nervous system can be thought of as a second motor control system, since much of the target tissues are smooth muscles of organs and viscera. The fine control of these numerous end organs is accomplished by usually two components of the autonomic nervous system acting in concert: the parasympathetic and sympathetic systems. More than 75% of parasympathetic nerve projections (not shown) take their origin from the vagal nerves (cranial nerve X). These projections exit the brain high in the neck, and splay out down through the body in branches, both rostrally and caudally, to innervate their target tissues. The neurons that give rise to the sympathetic branches of the autonomic nervous system are found in the ventromedial horn of gray matter at each vertebral level from T1–L2. This is shown in the diagram of the brain and cord to the *right*.

to less than one vertebral segment of the cord in its extent (Tuszynski et al. 1999; Bunge et al. 1993). Furthermore, within a matter of hours after the injury, sometimes even days, most of the neural machinery above and below the lesion remains intact. This state does not persist for long, however, as the injury to single cells and their processes progressively worsen, leading to cell death in the gray matter, and secondary axotomy and Wallerian degeneration in the white matter. These latter terms describe the slow dissolution of a local region of a single nerve fiber until it breaks into two pieces, followed by the complete autolytic destruction of the distal segment (that part of the fiber separated from the neuron's cell body) by the immune system. Such progressive destruction, or dying back, of the process that has survived injury seem curious. It is certainly unique and distinct from both programmed cell death (apoptosis) or Wallerian degeneration. This topic will be addressed again later in this monograph (see Chap. 7, Sect. 7.3, "Regeneration"). For an informative review of cell and cell process death in the nervous system, refer to Raff et al. (2002). The loss of the distal segment of the nerve fiber was described by Augustus Volney Waller in 1850, hence the name Wallerian degeneration.

In summary, I emphasize that (a) spinal cord injuries in humans are reasonably localized; (b) the destruction of gray matter and its neurons are *not* significantly associated with the catastrophic behavioral loss observed after SCI; (c) the localized interruption in the long communication circuits between body and brain contained within the spinal cord white matter is central to the behavioral loss after SCI, and (d) this disconnect leads to a permanent condition of motor and sensory loss, the permanent loss of their distal segments, and the nonfunctional status of white matter tracts surviving the injury.

To make these points, I have not discussed the other types of cells of the spinal cord that play a role in the injury. These include interneurons that far outnumber the other types of nerve cells in gray matter, the glia (astrocytes and oligodendrocytes), microglia, and numerous types of cell immigrants entering the spinal cord wound from the peripheral environment such as Schwann cells, fibroblasts, macrophages and other blood-borne cells. These all will come up in particular discussions to follow.

These sympathetic projections are organized as sympathetic ganglia (the paravertebral ganglia) that are bilaterally organized; only the left side is shown for diagrammatic purpose. The general regions of the body innervated by the sympathetic nerves projecting from these ganglia are *color-coded* in the human form to the *left*. Note that a spinal cord injury above T1 isolates the neurons and projections of the sympathetic system from the parasympathetic system, which leaves major functioning of one system unopposed by the other. A clinical manifestation of such compartmentalization of the autonomic nervous system can be seen in the dangerous clinical condition, autonomic dysreflexia, sometimes associated with quadriplegia. In this syndrome, a minor sensory stimulus can activate sympathetic discharge to the heart and vascular system unopposed by descending parasympathetic inhibition. The symptoms of spiking unregulated blood pressure can cause cerebral aneurysms and even death

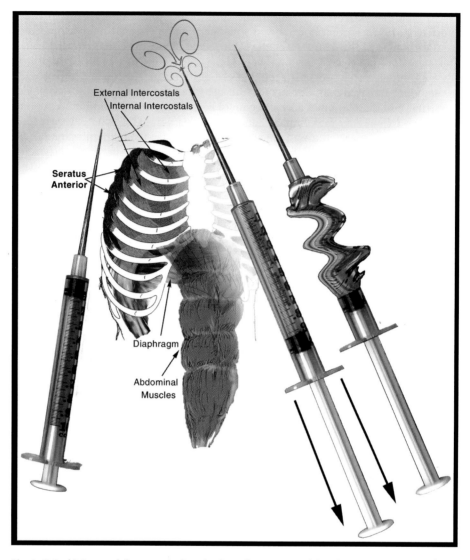

Fig. 6. Spinal injury and the control of respiration. The anatomy of the rib cage is illustrated, and in *colors*, the intercostal muscles (external and the internal intercostals, lying underneath), which control the movement of the rib cage during inspiration and expiration are shown. The location of the primary organ of respiration, the diaphragm, is shown, as is the abdominal musculature and additional accessory musculature that play a role in the respiratory cycle. It is both convenient and instructive to consider the pleural cavity as a syringe (*far left*), the stiff wall of the syringe, by analogy, to the wall of the pleural cavity, the rigidity of its architecture controlled by intercostal muscles. Next, to the *right*, the plunger of the syringe is pulled down, pulling air into the syringe from the orifice of the needle. This plunger, by analogy, represents the muscular contraction of the diaphragm. To the *far right*, the consequence of making the wall of the syringe weak and flimsy is shown, causing it to collapse when the plunger is pulled back, preventing much air from being drawn into the syringe. This is similar to the consequence of upper thoracic (and higher) SCI, where control of the intercostals and accessory musculature is lost. Rigidity of the rib cage is thus lost,

2.2.1
The Biological Basis of the Injury

I have emphasized that injury to the human brain and spinal cord leads to catastrophic life-long behavioral loss. This failure to repair injury to the CNS is known to be due in large part to the lack of sustained nerve regeneration, followed by the formation of new functional synapses within the brain and spinal cord. Nerve fibers located in the trunk and extremities of mammals (the peripheral nervous system, or PNS) in fact do regenerate following severe injury – sometimes reestablishing functional synapses with so-called end organs (for example, muscle fibers or sensory receptors). These naturally formed neural connections are associated with variable levels of functional recovery (Thomas 1988; Fawcett and Keynes 1990; Ketchum 1982; Freed et al. 1985).

Curiously, mammalian nerve processes projecting from a bipolar dorsal root ganglion neuron into a limb, regenerate with facility since they are outside the environment of the brain and spinal cord. The other process from the same cell projecting into the spinal cord does not regenerate, ostensibly because it is located within the environment of the CNS. This paradox, as most of the confounding aspects of CNS and PNS regeneration, were first systematically evaluated by the Nobel laureate, Santiago Ramón y Cajal, in the latter part of the nineteenth century. His two-volume treatise *Degeneration and Regeneration of the Nervous System*, completed just after the turn of the nineteenth century, and published in English in 1928, is still worthwhile reading for students of CNS trauma. Since the publication of Ramón y Cajal's book, it has been recognized that any technology that both facilitates and directs nerve regeneration in the brain or spinal cord would be of incalculable therapeutic value.

The notion that axonal regeneration within the spinal cord may correct for the behavioral deficits produced by severe injury is rooted in the observation that mammals, and perhaps birds, nearly stand alone in the world of vertebrates as creatures that do not regenerate their spinal cord nerve processes (Chernoff 1995). Spinal cord regeneration leading to various degrees of functional recovery is characteristic of primitive cartilaginous fish (Rovainen 1967; Wood and Cohen 1979; Borgens 1981) as well as modern bony fish (Bernstein et al. 1978; Bernstein and Bernstein 1967; Anderson et al. 1983), amphibians (Singer et al. 1979), reptiles (Simpson 1968; Duffy et al. 1992), the tadpoles of frogs and toads (Beattie et al. 1990), during fetal development of birds and mammals (Shimizu et al. 1990; Iwashita et al. 1994), and in some species of immature mammals such as opossum, while they are still in the marsupium of the mother (Treherne 1992).

There is at least one important lesson to be gleaned from the literature on comparative spinal cord regeneration. For functional recovery to be reestablished it is not required that point-to-point synaptic connections be restored. Inappropriate connec-

---

causing flail chest syndrome. This can contribute to poor respiratory control even if innervation to the diaphragm survives the spinal injury, or in quadriplegics when the diaphragm is artificially paced using a phrenic stimulator

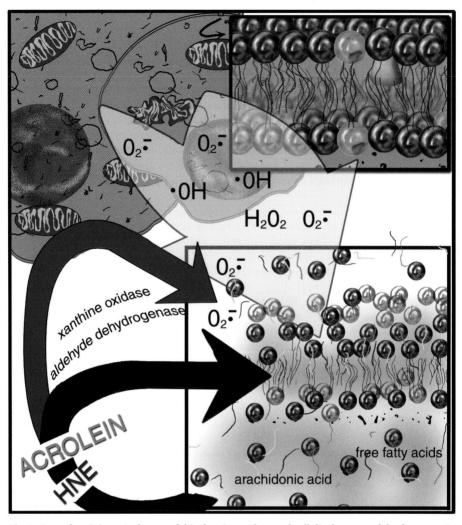

Fig. 7. Secondary injury. At the *top* of this drawing, a damaged cell displays one of the first steps in the secondary injury phenomenon: collapse of the mitochondria and their oxidative metabolism. This leads to the an overproduction of several so-called free radicals, which are highly reactive oxygen metabolites; super oxide (O_2^-) in particular, as well as hydroxyl ions (*OH*) and hydrogen peroxide (H_2O_2). These highly reactive species destroy the integrity of cell membranes, releasing free fatty acids; one of most damaging products is arachidonic acid. Continuing peroxidation of these free membrane lipids generates products such as acrolein and 4-hydroxynonenal (*HNE*), both of which are very toxic. These in turn feed back to destroy more cell membrane, releasing yet more free fatty acids to undergo lipid peroxidation in an autocatalytic process of self-destruction, not only for the cells that were originally damaged, but for nearby undamaged cells as well. Enzymes such as xanthanine oxidase also use acrolein as a substrate to produce more super oxide radicals in another positive feedback pathway leading to more membrane breakdown. The collapse of oxidative metabolism by mitochondria, the production of free radicals, and lipid peroxidation are the molecular bases for secondary injury in the CNS

tions can still subserve appropriate behavioral recovery. It is also the take home message – often not emphasized – of more modern techniques applied to mammals claiming functional recovery secondary to facilitated regeneration after CNS trauma. I do not know of one experimental procedure in the mammal even claiming to reestablish appropriate connections in the spinal cord in number or kind – even though a seemingly appropriate functional recovery of specific behaviors is reported. It is likely that a small number of inappropriate synapses formed just on either side of the lesion may be sufficient to reproduce a functional behavioral repertoire as observed in the goldfish and ammocoete lamprey. The mechanisms underlying the expression of appropriate behaviors subsequent to such short distance axonal regeneration are yet to be understood. This state of ignorance will likely continue on into the future for several reasons, chief among which is the paucity of experimental techniques that can induce significant axonal regeneration leading to a true behavioral recovery. This model still awaits us, and is required to unravel this mystery in the mammal. The whole issue of CNS behavioral recovery is indeed both murky, but challenging. Often, functional behaviors that reappear after spinal cord injury are really facsimiles. To balance one's thinking on these issues, the now dated, but still informative discussion by Michael Goldberger and Marion Murray in 1978 should be required reading. Their discussion centered on chronic deafferentation of spinal circuits began with the heading "In Recovery, What Is Recovered?"

2.2.2
Secondary Injury

Steady, progressive loss of axons and neurons after impact to the cord is a hallmark of SCI, often referred to as secondary injury. This term notes a distinct phase of progressive destruction of spinal cord tissue following the immediate consequences of the impact to CNS tissue (the primary injury). This wave of destruction can occur over many days, even weeks. It is autocatalytic, self-propagating, and involves numerous biological processes and biochemistries. Secondary injury is initiated by damage to the cell membrane – breaking its ionic seal. Ionic derangement is the result, that is, the mixing of ions across the membrane. This membrane normally acts to segregate ion species to the intracellular and extracellular compartments.

Ionic derangement is the earliest pathology critical to progressive destruction of the spinal cord. Ionic derangement is sometimes referred to as occult damage because this insult is hidden from view and mysterious. The prime villain appears to be poorly regulated, or unregulated entry of Ca^{++} into neurons or local regions of damaged axons (Borgens 1988; Honou and Young 1995; Lee et al. 1999; Maxwell 1996). Increases in cytoplasmic Ca^{++} likely induce most of the key pathologies associated with secondary injury. For example, it has been known for over 30 years that increases in cytosolic Ca^{++} destabilize the cytoskeleton, indeed depolymerize tubulins, degrade microfilaments, destabilize the integrity of the membrane itself, and shut down axoplasmic transport. Experiments by William Schlaepfer, later aided by his colleague Richard Bunge, nailed this proposition over 30 years ago. This includes the classic demonstration that a cuff placed around a peripheral nerve and impregnated with the Ca^{++} ionophore A23187, induced a localized dissolution of the nerve trunk underneath it (Schlaepfer 1974, 1977).

Unregulated spikes in cytosolic Ca^{++} are aided by increases in intracellular Na^+ (moving down its electrochemical gradient into the cell as well). Na^+ increase in cytoplasm initiates release of Ca^{++} from intracellular stores such as mitochondria, and the liberation of bound cytosolic Ca^{++} in self-reinforcing positive feedback (Carafoli and Crompton 1976). Elevated levels of Ca^{++} ions in the cytoplasm up-regulate normally quiescent (or low) activity of catabolic enzymes such as caspases, cysteine proteases, phospholipases, and key enzymes associated with the induction of apoptosis. When intra-axonal concentrations of Na^+ increase above the physiological level, the action of the Na^+/Ca^{++} exchanger in the membrane may work in the reverse from normal. That is, after injury, Ca^{++} is pumped inwards while Na^+ is extruded from the cytoplasm (Stys 1992, 1998; Stys et al. 1992). There is also a Na^+/Ca^{++} exchanger in mitochondrial membranes, exchanging one ion for another. Mitochondrial exchangers normally extrude Na^+ while taking up Ca^{++} (remember that mitochondria are calcium reservoirs within the cell). An increase in cytosolic Ca^{++} produced by injury to the cell will likely push this exchanger to work in reverse, causing it to extrude Ca^{++} from mitochondria back into the cytoplasmic compartment. One can begin to appreciate that after mechanical damage to neurons and/or their axons, everything that can go wrong with Ca^{++} homeostasis does, with the net result of increased intracellular Ca^{++} and its extremely damaging consequences. One last point on this topic: remember the movement of water accompanies Na^+ transport. The increase in Na^+ movement into organelles, as occurs in mitochondria, is likely responsible for their swelling and bursting under pathological conditions (Trump et al. 1988).

Since spinal cord injury is a hemorrhagic injury, glucose and oxygen deprivation contribute substantially to continuing destruction of the tissue during the secondary injury phase. Ischemia is a direct contributor to dissolution of the parenchyma, just as in head injury or stroke. Incomplete oxygen metabolism within the cell, coupled with specific enzymatic catalysis, leads to the formation of highly reactive oxygen species such as superoxide anion, hydrogen peroxide, and hydroxy radicals, the so called free radicals (or better yet, reactive oxygen intermediates). These compounds are also cytodestructive and contribute to the increasing mechanisms of cell and tissue destruction directly, or secondarily, by promoting lipid peroxidation. Metabolites of arachidonic acid like thromboxanes and leukotrienes impact inflammation and vascular perfusion of the injury. This biochemistry is complex, and many other byproducts of lipid peroxidation such as acrolein, are known cellular toxins (Fig. 7). The production of some endogenous antioxidants are reduced by SCI reflecting continuing oxidative processes that are part of the injury process – but may also reduce the level of neuroprotection afforded spinal cord tissue (Pietronigro et al. 1983, 1985; Lemke et al. 1990; Azbill et al. 1997).

Derangement in oxygen levels, glucose, and Ca^{++} metabolism is further exacerbated by reperfusion injury, the injury to cells associated with the reintroduction of isotonic fluids and a return of normal oxygen tension (Kim-Lee et al. 1992). For example, the ability of acrolein to interfere with or destroy compound action potential conduction in isolated spinal cords has been thoroughly examined in a reperfusion model. Nerve impulse conduction through normal white matter maintained under normal conditions in organ culture is not affected by 50 μM acrolein in the bathing media, but reversibly compromised by 200 μM. After 1 h of oxygen and glucose deprivation, and a return to a normal media, 50 μM acrolein dramatically compromised conduction, and 200 μM irreversibly kills it (Peasley et al., unpublished observations). At the tissue level, the swelling of the cord, the formation of cysts and syrinxes (swollen central canal) and likely autoimmune reactions, which are still poorly understood, all interact in the secondary injury phase of SCI.

2.2.3
Acute and Chronic Phases of SCI Can Be Considered Two Separate Injuries

In the common vernacular of the trauma clinic, acute refers to fresh injuries or those of sudden onset. Chronic refers to a long-standing injury. Actually, it is not possible to ascribe a time after injury where the acute phase grades into the chronic phase. Certainly within hours, even a few days after an injury, "acute" seems correct in usage, while months to years after injury is reasonably characterized as a chronic injury. Though the progression of pathology in every spinal cord injury is variable in character, these terms, though imprecise, have utility. In recent years the term "subacute" has been used to bridge these two phases of the injury.

While the actual periods of time may be imprecise, the biology of the acute and chronic phases are distinctly different. So much so, that with regard to experimental therapies aimed at improving functional recovery, they may as well be treated as separate types of injury.

Simply put, in the stable chronic SCI, substantial anatomy has been irreversibly lost. The distal axonal segments of significant portions of white matter tracts have degenerated, and in some cases induce degenerative changes in their target neurons or muscle cells. Consider this further. In a truly chronic injury, the axons of whole columns of ascending white matter tracts rostral to the injury are no longer there. On the caudal side of the injury, entire columns of descending tracts are simply not there – the axons long since having undergone Wallerian degeneration. Most of the central core of the cord within the vertebral segment of injury – mostly gray matter – in addition to variable amounts of white matter, is indeed destroyed. The loss of this sometimes substantial volume of spinal cord tissue can produce a stenotic, hour glass-shaped zone of injury (see Moriarty et al. 1998; Duerstock and Borgens 2000).

The region formerly occupied by both gray and white matter is replaced by scar tissue in the chronic phase of spinal cord injury. Spinal scar is of a complex origin. Typically, collagen producing fibroblasts migrate into the lesion, especially where the dura is compromised, suggesting fibroblasts from adjacent bone and muscle are the source of this immigration (Krikorian et al. 1981). Together with the explosive increase in astrocytes (glial hyperplasia), these cells and their extracellular matrix form a dense mat. This scar is often referred to as the fibroglial scar, denoting its dual cellular origin. A new basal lamina is formed at the boundary of the CNS/PNS environment in an attempt by cells to once again seal and separate the CNS and PNS compartments. This basal lamina is subtended by a glial limitans, a secondary sheath produced by the interlocked end feet of astrocytes. The components of this cicatrix plus the bounding laminae have been considered a physical barrier to nerve regeneration for over 100 years (reviewed by Reier et al. 1983); however, after 100 years of debate, this interpretation is still untenable.

3 The Scar as a Barrier to Regeneration

Many pioneers in SCI research of the 1950s such as William Windle and Carmine Clemente strongly believed the physical barrier hypothesis early in their careers. Furthermore, they believed the claims of axonal regeneration in adult mammals after administration of pyromen (a bacterial polysaccharide), corticoids, a variety of enzyme treatments, and precise surgery was due to a partial dissolution of the fibroglial scar. The beginning of the demise of the physical barrier hypothesis came from two sources a decade later: (1) the lack of consensus that axonal regeneration was actually enhanced by the above techniques (i.e., a failure of others to repeat these experiments), and (2) the comparative anatomy of spinal cord regeneration, particularly in teleost fish. The classic experiments of Gerald and Mary Bernstein (Bernstein 1978; Bernstein and Bernstein 1967) using goldfish that possess native powers of spinal cord regeneration should be brought to mind. They demonstrated that a dense scar indeed forms at the site of transection of the cord in goldfish. A sleeve of Teflon was inserted into the transection, which prevented axons from crossing this lesion, but did not affect the formation of the scar on either side. Subsequently, the Teflon sheet was removed and the cord was transected once again rostral to the original injury. Spinal cord axons regenerated through the first lesion and of course through the scar that developed there as well. The Bernsteins' further determined that Teflon deflected axons made synaptic connections without being able to cross the caudal segment of cord, raising the interesting possibility that this synapse formation halted further axonal advance (Bernstein and Bernstein 1971).

The scar barrier hypothesis cannot account for a variety of other observations either. First, it is well known that monoaminergic and adrenergic axons of the adult mammalian spinal cord regenerate with facility in certain conditions and through scar tissue (Bjorklund et al. 1971, 1972, 1973). Another type of CNS axon that regenerates in the adult mammal is neurosecretory axons. The proximal segments of neurohypophysial axons regenerate through scar tissue to form new synapses within the posterior lobe of the pituitary. Scar tissue formed after lesions to the hypothalamus and thalamus is just as impressive as that in spinal cord (see Kiernan 1979). Recent reports from Geoffery Raisman's laboratory in England continue to demonstrate that when CNS sprouting is induced near or within the lesion of the brain, that growth of axons occurs within and through the scar (Li and Raisman 1995).

Though it is likely that the CNS scar may not present a physical barrier to regeneration, it clearly seems inhospitable for the regeneration of (particularly) myelinated axons. This nonpermissive character is likely derived from at least three sources: (1) characteristics of the cells and their matrix, which may deflect or confuse axonal growth, (2) astrocytes may provide a physiological stop signal to growing nerve processes when they contact this class of glial cell (Liuzzi and Lasek 1987), and (3) the presence of inhibitory molecules associated with the membranes of glial cells.

3.1
Inhibitory Molecules

Hypotheses relating physical barriers and a lack of trophic (nutritive) and tropic (guidance) factors have dominated theories of the lack of regeneration of the CNS for most of the last one and a half centuries. That evolution might select for factors that are inhibitory to regeneration of mammalian brain and spinal cord tissues seemed illogical given the powers of regeneration observed in the CNS of many non-mammalian vertebrates. Ramón y Cajal (1928), once again: *"It may also be inferred that this defective capacity for regeneration does not depend on essential, fatal, and unchangeable conditions, but on the absence in the surroundings of catalytic agents able to overcome the osmotic equilibria of the cones of growth to provoke their vigorous nutrition and to direct them to the path that they must follow"* (1928, p 744).

Modern investigators such as Martin Berry have predicted the phenomenon of active central inhibition of axonal regeneration for decades (McConnell and Berry 1982). More recently, the first inhibitory factors to be identified and characterized (NI-250, a complex, likely containing NI-35) were associated with the membranes of CNS myelin-producing cells, the oligodendrocytes, (Caroni and Schwab 1988a) and a monoclonal antibody (IN-1) developed against them (Caroni and Schwab 1988b). This was an important achievement in unraveling the biological basis for abortive regeneration. We will revisit this topic again in Chap. 7, Sect. 7.3.4, "Inhibiting the Inhibitors of Nerve Regeneration", as a strategy for facilitating spinal cord regeneration; however, it is wise to point out that in spite of the universal acceptance of this hypothesis of a central myelin inhibition of regeneration, there are numerous experiments that fail to support the contribution of myelin-associated protein, degenerating myelin, or generally, CNS glia, to the collapse of regenerative growth in the spinal cord of the adult mammal (see Davies et al. 1997, 1999; Berry et al. 1992 for samples and discussion).

3.1.1
Other Inhibitors

There are other biochemistries and molecules that likely play a role in the inhibition of regeneration associated with the fibroglial scar, and their number seems to grow every year. Molecules that clearly induce growth cone collapse in embryonic models, in vitro studies, and CNS injury models include the semaphorins, versican, neurocan, and brevican (all proteoglycans), and the well-known adhesivity factor, tenascin (Miranda et al. 1999; Reza et al. 1999; Fawcett and Asher 1999; Pasterkamp 1998). Furthermore, astrocytes increase in number explosively after spinal cord injury, not oligodendrocytes. On the basis of cell density alone, these cells are most likely to play a key role in inhibiting the growth of axons. Further, as if things were not complicated enough, it is wise to remember that glia produce a variety of factors which are also supportive or facilitative of axonal regeneration. For example, ciliary neurotrophic factor (CNTF), a potent neuroprotective molecule, is up-regulated in reactive astrocytes of the injured adult rat spinal cord (Lee et al. 1998).

Personally, it has always made more sense to me that the astrocyte is the critical mediator of regeneration, or the lack thereof, within the spinal cord scar of the mammal. That is the lesson of the historical literature. Recently, Jerry Silver's laboratory has explored these old issues once again with a creative and novel new technology. They used transgenic mice expressing green fluorescent protein (GFP) in their tissues as donors for nervous tissue that was later implanted into rats. (They actually select their green donor mice using a black light.) This graft results in unambiguous identification of the origin of regenerating axons and sprouts (which are naturally fluorescent) in various different experimental contexts. They have reported that green sensory ganglia transplanted into both cord or brain regenerated axons extensive distances through normal white matter (apparently undamaged), degenerating white matter, and even through scar tissue. Near the center of mature scar, axons were deflected, but not because of physical barriers. The turning or collapse of growth cones was associated with increasing concentrations of proteoglycan matrix molecules of chondroitin sulfate, a secretion product of astrocytes and other cells such as macrophages (Davies et al. 1999; Fitch and Silver 1997). Furthermore, axonal regeneration was not inhibited by all reactive astrocytes (identified immunocytochemically), suggesting at least two populations of glial cells arise after activation by injury. At least one of these groups is inhibitory to CNS nerve regeneration, while the other may facilitate axonal growth and sprouting. So far their conclusions provide the best compromise between the older and newer literature on the inhibitory contribution of scar tissue.

Silver and colleagues comment on the likely minor role of myelin-associated proteins and oligodendrocytes in the overall scheme of the abortive regeneration of axons in mammalian spinal cord. The growth of axons into regions of normal and degenerate white matter *"appear not to be in a struggle with the environment that must surely contain large compliments of purportedly potent myelin-associated inhibitors..."* (Davies et al. 1999, p 5818). They also instruct that the clear inhibitory effects of myelin, associated protein on nerve growth in vitro, can be reversed by the presence of astrocytes (Fawcett et al. 1992). We should remember, however, that this test vehicle was a xenograft of genetically engineered cells.

Martin Berry, a fellow with a long history of clever experimentation, tested the proposed inhibition of CNS myelin-associated protein in another way. Oligodendrocytes and CNS myelin are absent from the proximal portion of the optic nerve of the Browman-Wise mutant rat. Thus, one should expect that in the absence of potent inhibitory factors associated with CNS myelin (or the oligodendrocytes), optic nerve axons would regenerate with facility; however, they did not. In other mutants, optic nerve axons regenerated readily in association with Schwann cell tubes, an unnatural inhabitant of the optic nerve in these mutant animals, but the axons abruptly stopped growing at the end of the tube. This particular report (Berry et al. 1992) has an interesting and helpful discussion concerning the confused state of both oligodendrocytes and astrocytes in the grand schemes of axonal inhibition by glia of the mammalian CNS. Still, my reading of this broad literature suggests that strategies of inhibition harken back to the older literature where the astrocyte has always been viewed as the culprit rather than the oligodendrocyte (reviewed by Reier et al. 1983).

Astrocytes likely possess their own membrane-bound inhibitory molecules analogous to IN-250 and -35. After injury, activated astrocytes up-regulate glial fibrillary acidic protein (GFAP) and another membrane protein, rTAPA (target of the antiproliferative antibody). The latter appears as a good candidate for an astrocyte inhibitory factor (Geisert et al. 1996).

Close by in the lesion, the neurons of gray matter up-regulate significant amounts of other potent signaling molecules or nerve growth factors, particularly members of the neurotrophin gene family such as brain-derived neurotrophic factor (BDNF), neurotrophin 3 and 4/5. It is clear that the balance between the up-regulation of inhibitory and facilitative biochemistries in injured mammalian CNS is deeply complicated, and the interactions extraordinarily subtle. For example, exposure of the nerve growth cone to a neurotrophin may completely switch the response of the cell to other signaling molecules. What was before exposure an inhibitory influence (i.e., to myelin-associated protein) becomes a positive guidance cue after exposure to the neurotrophin (Cai et al. 1999; see also Song and Poo 1999).

In spite of these important, contradictory, sometimes vexatious, observations, it is my opinion that when a particularly robust means of initiating axonal regeneration within the cord is provided to the proximal segments of CNS axons, they will likely penetrate scar tissue in spite of these obstacles. We have studied axons regenerating into mature glial scar of transected spinal cords of adult guinea pigs induced by electrical fields (see Chap. 11, Sect. 11.2, "The Anatomy of Regeneration of Spinal Cord Nerve Fibers in the Laboratory Rat and Guinea Pig" and Sect. 11.3, "Guiding Spinal Cord Axons into Rubber Tubes with Applied Voltages"). Three-dimensional reconstruction of confocal images revealed that ascending axons were able to penetrate the scar to enter the rostral segment of cord (Borgens and Bohnert 1997; and Borgens 1999). Such axon penetrations of scar do not occur in sham-treated animals. Mature cartilage is considered extremely nonpermissive to axon penetration, in part because of its dense physical nature and its composition: it contains high concentrations of nonpermissive chondroitin sulfates. Over 20 years ago, we demonstrated that the cartilage core of hypomorphically regenerating adult *Xenopus* limbs could indeed be penetrated by regenerating peripheral axons (Borgens et al. 1979).

3.2
Other Cells Important to SCI

Other important anatomical characteristics of the chronic phase of the injury include the spared, but nonfunctional rind of white matter, hypervascularity in the region of the injury (Blight 1991), and sometimes extensive cavitation of the spinal cord. Cavitations likely result from the action of phagocytes that are "doing their job" cleaning up the wound. There is an extensive migration of macrophages into the injury during the acute phase, producing what has been called bystander damage (Fig. 8; Blight 1985; Moriarity et al. 1998; Leskovar 2000). Transformation of CNS microglia into macrophages also occurs, but these cells play a lesser role in phagocytosis, dominated as they are by the number of invading macrophages of myelomonocytic lineage. There are two theories concerning this invasion of phagocytes. One notion is that the massive numbers of macrophages moving into the spinal wound kill other cells (bystander damage) and create an acidic, catabolic environment that contributes to

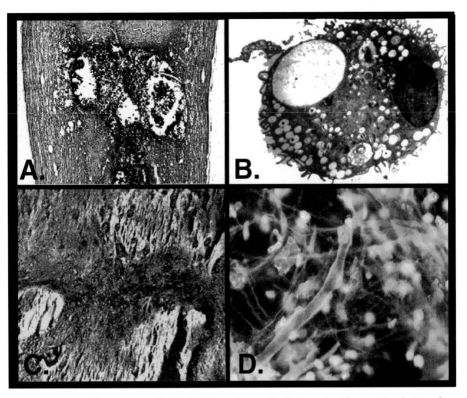

Fig. 8A–D. Macrophages. In **A**, the dark T-shaped mass is the 3-week-old contusion lesion of rat thoracic spinal cord inundated with macrophages. The dark stain is due to the use of a monoclonal antibody specific for activated macrophages, labeling the thousands that occupy the site of spinal cord damage. In **B**, an electron photomicrograph of an activated macrophage, the large vesicles and vacuoles are characteristic of these active phagocytes, many times filled with portions of erythrocytes and cell debris. This cell was approximately 12 µm in diameter and typical of the macrophages found in acute CNS wounds. Macrophages are extremely mobile. Most that occupy the spinal lesion are of myelomonocytic lineage, entering the damaged region from its vascular supply. A small number of macrophages arise from transformation of resident microglia. A few microliters of a rhodamine dextran can be a reasonably effective macrophage marker since it is imbibed by these phagocytes or bonds to their sticky surface. While this is not a highly specific means of macrophage identification, it does show the large numbers of these mobile phagocytes that migrate into the lesion from far away. The label was injected about 3 mm from the site of the lesion shown in **C**. The *red speckles* are mostly macrophages that migrated into the lesion, shown in the loose stroma of this fresh injury at a higher magnification in D

progressive dissolution of the spinal cord tissues. As well, macrophages crossing the blood–brain barrier during the stage of inflammation may be associated with increases in potent inhibitory extracellular matrix molecules such as certain families of proteoglycans (Fitch and Silver 1997) and the release of potent cytokines such as interleukin 1 and tumor necrosis factor β(IL-1, and TNF-β; Leskovar et al. 2000), that enhance scarring and neoangiogenesis. Administration of macrophage toxins such as silica is associated with an improved recovery from spinal cord and cerebral damage, which supports this notion (Blight 1994 and Giulian et al. 1989). The alternative suggestion is that macrophages confer special properties to the healthy axons in their surroundings, leading to regeneration (such as normally occurs in the peripheral nervous system). In contrast, this notion holds that the late arrival of reduced numbers of macrophages in spinal lesions (relative to peripheral nerve injuries) contributes to the failure of regeneration in the CNS (Perry and Brown 1992; Perry and Gordon 1988, 1991; Perry et al. 1993). This is supported by the fact that transplants of additional macrophages, activated in peripheral wounds, produce regeneration of CNS axons in optic nerves (Lazarov-Spiegler et al. 1996). I hold for the bystander damage notion and will discuss this issue more in Chap. 7, Sect. 7.3.5, "Do Macrophages Hurt or Help Regeneration in the Spinal Cord?", since a clinical therapy has recently begun based on transplantation of macrophages into human spinal injuries.

Schwann cells (also immigrants to the lesion) and astrocytes are also known to phagocytose dead and dying cells. The cavitation produced by all of these cells may coalesce with the sometimes extensive swelling of the central canal. Clinically, the large cysts (likely products of hemorrhagic necrosis and phagocytosis) compress healthy cord by swelling from the inside. These cysts are associated with complicated neuropathies, including altered pressure gradients within the CSF and mechanical distension of the spinal cord, especially when it is "tethered" (Greitz et al. 1999). Large cysts are usually drained by surgical techniques and are a cause of rehospitalization for chronically injured patients.

4 Treating the Acute and Chronic Injury: Historical Perspective

Most of the early work directed towards new clinical therapies focused on the issue of the mature fibroglial scar, and ways to alter its extent and density.

The first exogenous substance claimed to produce axonal regeneration in the adult mammalian spinal cord was pyromen, a pyrogenic polysaccharide derived from bacteria. This first exciting report by William Windle and William Chambers, soon after the end of WWII in 1950, ushered in an era of optimism concerning clinical possibilities for SCI, born of experimental biology. Parenterally administered pyromen was known to induce the secretion of growth-associated substances (somatotrophins) and anti-inflammatory substances (such as the corticotrophins and adrenal corticosteroids) from the adenohypophysis and adrenocorticotrophic hormone (ACTH) directly from the pituitary. The latter hypothalamic/ACTH/pituitary axis response to pyromen indicated that inflammation and scar tissue at the spinal lesion should be ameliorated. The histological responses to Pyromen indicated that the scar tissue in spinal lesions (Clemente 1955) and later in brain (Fertig et al. 1971) was indeed altered, particularly in its fibrous component (see reviews by Windle 1956; Clemente 1964). Unfortunately, as Martin Berry (1979) colorfully exclaimed, *"this Indian summer of hope was short-lived as negative results began to appear in the literature"* (p 77). Indeed, the late 1950s to the early 1970s were marked by controversy over the effects of pyromen. Its effects on regeneration and on scar tissue could not be confirmed by numerous laboratories (Lance 1954; Areta 1956; O'Callaghan and Speakman 1963). Martin Berry, again... *"the results with Pyromen, although initially so promising, were difficult to reproduce and it is perhaps significant that the drug never became established in the treatment of human paraplegia"* (Berry 1979, p 77).

Stemming in part from the early positive reports of pyromen, excitement in the popular and scientific literature was later stirred by a two Armenian investigators, L. Mantinian and A. Andreasian. These investigators claimed spinal cord regeneration in response to the administration of a cocktail of catabolic enzymes (hyaluronidase, trypsin, and elastase) designed to render the scar less of a barrier to regeneration. This Indian summer also collapsed through the failure to repeat or confirm the experiments, particularly by Lloyd Guth's laboratory (Guth et al. 1978) and Martin Berry (Knowles and Berry 1978; reviewed by Kiernan 1979), and the widely held notion that the seminal results were due to incomplete transection of the spinal cord.

Sometimes we, in science, throw out the baby with the bath water. The issue of the contribution of the scar to the failure of axonal regeneration is still as much alive today as 40 years ago, only now as an annotated exercise in biochemistry. I believe some of the enzymes and their combinations may still be useful tools to explore these issues and as a possible adjunct to the treatment regimens aimed at reducing inflammation and facilitating nerve regeneration.

Cooling the spinal cord by up to 10°C (hypothermia) during the acute phase is generally believed to reduce swelling, increase tolerance to the lack of oxygen (hypoxia), and hypothetically, reduce the level of hemorrhagic necrosis of spinal cord stressed by glucose and oxygen deprivation. The reduction of the temperature of the spinal cord at the site of injury in human patients sometimes involved wrapping a collar around the surgically exposed cord and running cold water through it or perfusion with cold sterile salines. This is not at all a trivial undertaking, as this region is very fragile, and the potential for injuring the spinal cord further is not so remote. A criticism of this early experimentation (see Albin et al. 1969; White et al. 1969) was indeed a concern for increased mortality due to such heroic methods. Other neurosurgeons believed that it was less the cooling of the spinal cord that may have been beneficial to patients, but the perfusions. The perfusions might have washed out many of the offending endogenous substances causing secondary injury (Tator and Deecke 1972).

More recent examples of acute interventions include:

1. The use of methylprednisolone (MP) (Bracken et al. 1990) was based less on its known propensity to reduce swelling, but rather its perceived ability to reduce free radical-mediated damage in the spinal cord of experimental animals. Initially, there were heightened expectations since MP was the first new treatment for acute spinal injury derived from animal studies (Hall 1992; Bracken et al. 1984). The first large, randomized, multicenter trials of SCI therapies (primarily MP) were called the National Acute Spinal Cord Injury Studies (NASCIS). NASCIS I failed to demonstrate the effectiveness of MP administration (Bracken et al. 1984, 1985). In the NASCIS II study, higher dosages of MP were claimed to improve motor functions by 6-month and 1-year checkups (Bracken et al. 1990, 1993). NASCIS III revealed a continued rational for MP administration after acute SCI, particularly by extending the time course of the therapy (Bracken et al. 1997,1998). The steroid should be administered within 8 h of the injury, and a delayed treatment was associated with even a worse functional outcome relative to controls (Bracken and Holford 1993). This therapy is still controversial. It should be pointed out that the excitement of the 1980s over new insights into the free radical contribution to secondary injury overshadowed another, more conservative literature concerned with glucocorticoid administration in brain injury and ischemia. In an important 1985 report published in *Science* by Robert Sapolsky and William Pulsenelli, the authors reviewed the damaging effects of glucocorticoid administration in CNS ischemia, discussing a larger literature suggesting that nerve survival in general is compromised by steroids, especially when they are exposed to known endotoxins such as kainic acid (known to be present after SCI). Additionally, many neurosurgeons have been unimpressed with the modest to undetectable level of improvement in their patients. However, they have been impressed with heightened susceptibility to pneumonia and urinary tract infections associated with this treatment. Overall, the claimed marginal results balanced against the hazards of MP use, and problems inherent in the statistics used to evaluate the clinical trials, has been recently reconsidered (Short et al. 2000; Pointillant et al. 2000; Nesathurai 2000).

2. The health concerns associated with massive glucocorticoid administration led to consideration of alternative drugs – also potent free radical scavengers – the 21 aminosteroids. These compounds (called lazaroids) are synthetic nonglucocorticoid steroids, which, unlike methylprednisolone, apparently do not cause significant immunosuppression or hypoglycemia, while preserving tissue concentrations of natural antioxidants such as vitamin E. One of these, tirilazid mesylate, was included for testing in NASCIS II but did not show efficiency at the dosages used.

3. A more esoteric notion relevant to the acute stage of spinal injury relates to the possible role of endogenous opioids during the phase of secondary injury. Opioids exert their effect on cells through receptor-mediated modes of action. The opiate receptor antagonist Naxolone, drew attention as a possible therapeutic agent; however, clinical trials in spinal injury failed to confirm any beneficial effect of Naxolone compared to placebo controls (Bracken et al. 1990).

4. Gangliosides are natural components of cell membranes. One of these glycolipids has been suggested as being instrumental during the development and regeneration of the nervous system. In the early 1980s, it had been claimed that administration of Ganglioside GM-1 (Sygen) promotes axonal regeneration and sprouting (see Wojcik et al. 1982; Sabel et al. 1988). Though the biological basis for the beneficial action of GM-1 is still unclear, it was administered to spinal cord-injured patients in a small clinical trial, where improvements in outcome were reported, and with an administration window of 24 h after injury (Geisler et al. 1991). The results of a large recently completed clinical trial however, did not support the long term usefulness of ganglioside therapy to spinal cord patients (Geisler 2001). Modest levels of recovery may be a result of GM-1 administration, but at present, the results of a large and completed clinical trial remain unpublished, with some details provided on the worldwide web (www.cureparalysis.org).

5. Two other unsuccessful SCI clinical trials of recent times also deserve mention: administration of thyroid-releasing hormone (TRH) (Pitts 1995) and the Ca^{++} blocker nimodipine (Petitjean et al. 1998)

6. Brief mention of two, likely premature, neurotransplantation pilot studies should be included here: the transplantation of olfactory ensheating cells (derived from the recipient) and peripheral activated macrophages. These will be discussed in subsequent sections 7.3.2 "Regeneration in Response to Neurotransplantation", and 7.3.5 "Do Macrophages Hurt of Help Regeneration in the Spinal Cord?"

7. The novel use of polymers to seal and protect axons and neurons from progressive dissolution has arisen in only the last 3 years. Phase I human clinical trials of these new methods are slated to begin in 2003.

8. Another regeneration therapy, regeneration of spinal cord axons in response to applied extracellular voltage gradients (oscillating field stimulation, or OFS) has shown promise during the acute phase of the injury (Borgens et al. 1987, 1990, 1993a, 1999), but for inexplicable reasons, not in the chronic phase in animal studies (Borgens et al. 1993b). Clinical trials of OFS applied to severe, acute cases of SCI in humans began in 2000. This technology, as well as polymer application after SCI, will also be examined in detail in Chap. 13, "From a Laboratory Tool to a Clinical Application," and Chap. 15 "Sealing the Breach in Cell Membranes with Hydrophilic Polymers."

5 Concerning Behavioral Models
for Spinal Cord Injury in Animals

A thoughtful consideration of the limits of animal models of SCI is critical to the movement of a promising technique into the surgical ward. It will likely surprise the reader to learn that the recovery of walking behavior (voluntary ambulation) has always been a controversial means of analysis of recovery from spinal injury in experimental animals – so I will start here first. We instinctively make the leap from paralysis in the animal to the lifelong paralysis endured by human spinal cord-injured patients. Most investigators still use some form of stepping or walking (Cheng et al. 1997; Basso et al. 1995) or related tests (Tator and Fehlings 1991) to evaluate functional recovery in small animal models of SCI. These models should act as behavioral indexes of white matter integrity and/or renewed nerve impulse conduction through the lesion if they are to indicate recovery from SCI – but do they?

5.1
When Walking Is Not Walking

Man is the only obligatory bipedal animal. Even the occasional bipedalism exhibited by various animals such as bears, and particularly primates, is a variant form of four-legged locomotion arising from the quadruped ground plan of physiology and anatomy. The side-to-side gait of the human is not the same as the effective bipedal rope walking gait in great apes, which evolved from an arboreal existence. Here, the extension of the legs during upright locomotion is angled one in front of the other (Napier 1967; Tardieu et al. 1993). The highly evolved upright walking in man is dominated by supraspinal control (that is, originating in the brain). It is not restricted to organized centers initiating voluntary walking, but in exquisitely evolved descending circuits required to maintain balance and erect posture as well as drive locomotion. Posture and locomotion in human bipedalism is dominated by descending projections of the dorsolateral system (corticospinal and corticorubrospinal tracts) and the ventromedial system (tectospinal, vestibulospinal, interstitiospinal, and reticulospinal tracts refer to Fig. 1). These projections terminate in different parts of the spinal cord – for example, the corticospinal tract terminates in regions of large motor neurons and in the zone of the spinal cord dominated by internuncial neurons (a.k.a. interneurons), which modify motor neuron activity. The rubrospinal tract terminates in intermediate zones of gray matter where neurons with short propriospinal fibers are located, particularly important in postural control.

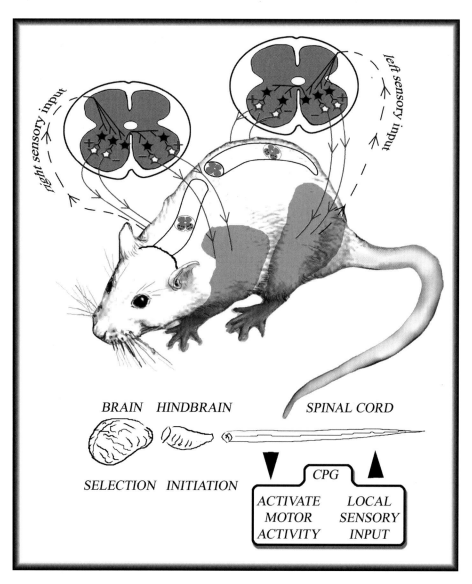

Fig. 9. Local reflex control of stepping in a spinal animal. The two diagrams of spinal cord segments provide some detail of the complexity of reflex circuits controlling muscle activity *at only that level of the spinal cord*. For ease of interpretation, only a schematic showing a reflex circuit dependent upon sensory input arising from the right side is shown on the "head end" of the spinal cord break. On the "tail side" of the spinal gap, only a circuit arising from sensory input from the left side is shown. Of course at each vertebral level of the cord – in the cervical and lumbosacral enlargements – such reflex circuitry is a mirror image on both sides of the cord's midline. This drawing is not representative of any one particular reflex (such as the myotactic, inverse myotactic, flexor withdrawal, etc.) but contains elements common to most spinal reflexes. First, the incoming sensory nerves (afferent signals) arise from specialized receptors in the joints, muscles, tendons, skin, etc. Specialized neurons (called interneurons, *black*) usually receive synapses from these sensory nerves entering the spinal cord at the dorsal root. Their fibers in turn project onto motorneurons (*red*) that

The problem for students of spinal cord paralysis is that in animals, voluntary walking is locally controlled and generated within the spinal cord, in sharp contrast to both the initiation and control of voluntary walking in man. The noted authority, Professor Anders Björkland, said it this way in his essay "A question of making it work" published in *Nature* in 1994: *"Then, as now, the main concern was that rats with a severed spinal cord could, unlike humans, regain mobility of their hindquarters"* (p 112).

In the four-legged animal, walking and stepping is initiated and performed by a combination of the reflex circuits localized to the spinal cord that communicate the functioning of a limb on one side of the body to the contralateral side by commissural axons that decussate within that spinal cord segment. These neural circuits coordinate opposite reflex behaviors such as the flexion of muscles of one limb coupled with the extension of the muscles of the other. The anatomy of spinal reflexes shows us that this agonist/antagonist machinery is available for use in stepping and gait. Reflex circuits and special neuronal modifier circuits called central pattern genera-

---

send their processes out of the ventral (anterior) spinal root to motor units within specific muscles on the same side of the body. The influence of the interneurons may be both to excite these motorneurons (and thus their corresponding muscles) or to inhibit them (diagrammed as the opposite sign). Ordinarily, on the same side of the body, excitation occurs in one group of muscles (i.e., the extensors of the limb) while the action of antagonistic muscles (the flexors) is inhibited on the other side of the body – and vice versa. Interneurons receiving sensory input from nerve fibers on one side of the midline send fibers to the other side (called commissural axons) that initiate antagonistic muscular contraction. This diagram is of course oversimplified. Some motorneurons receive direct input from incoming sensory fibers – and descending nerve fiber projections arising from the brain indeed modify motor neuron and interneuron behavior, usually by dampening it. There are several important points about spinal cord injury that can now be appreciated: First, reflex activity will be intact, and muscles will respond to sensory stimulation (such as the "tendon tap" reflex) below the level of even a complete spinal transection. Usually, reflex activity of the muscles below the spinal cord injury is actually *exaggerated* compared to normal because the "dampening" by descending projections from the brain is blocked at the injury. Second, it should be apparent that the "machinery" for considerable coordinated stepping and postural control can be controlled at the local level. While one limb undergoes complicated sets of activity – similar sets of muscles on the other side support this activity by performing opposite and/or complimentary functions through reciprocal innervation. This occurs independently in forelimbs *and* hindlimbs. The amount of coordinated and finely controlled stepping and gait that is locally controlled is impressive and supported by a further refinement of this basic ground plan. These are local neural circuits called central pattern generators (*CPGs*). The overall interaction between local sensory input and motor output as modified by CPGs is shown in the lower diagram. It is believed that *voluntary selection* of motor activity begins in the brain, which is initiated by *lower centers* in the brainstem. It is also believed that motor control by CPGs in the spinal cord is normally *inhibited* by descending neural projections arising from the brainstem from typically, reticulospinal neurons. Spinal cord injury then *disinhibits* the spinal centers of *four-legged animals*, allowing a more full expression of coordinated motor activity controlled at the level of the CPGs and bilateral reflex arcs. The result is a form of locomotion sometimes referred to as spinal stepping or walking. In humans, the disinhibition of lower motorneurons finds its expression in uncontrolled activation of limb musculature or spasticity. Moreover, the existence of CPGs in man is controversial – with the brainstem being more in command of the functions usually associated with CPGs in animals

tors (CPGs) (Fig. 9) work in concert to control locomotion. In quadruped animals, these neural circuits are localized within the relevant spinal cord segments associated with efferent (motor) and afferent (sensory) projections of the limbs. CPGs can generate complex patterns of rhythmic motor activity serving locomotion in animals in the complete absence of descending command signals from the brain. The actual motor activity of coordinated stepping and walking in four-legged animals is generated by CPGs. In lower vertebrates, such as the ammocoete lamprey, the cell biology and pharmacology of these circuits has been worked out (Grillner and Zangger 1979; Grillner et al. 1998), while much progress has been made in understanding the pharmacology/physiology of CPGs in the mammal (Kiehn et al. 1997). It is important to emphasize that CPG-mediated behaviors are neuromodulatory: they are adaptive and they respond to very subtle changes in sensory input by initiating very subtle changes in motor output (Marder and Calabrese 1996).

Are there CPGs in primates – particularly humans (Illis 1995)? CPG-mediated rhythmic motor output is very easy to elicit and record electrophysiologically in spinal nonprimate mammals by electrical or pharmacological stimulation. Over 20 years ago Eduardo Edilberg provided the first convincing evidence that something was quite amiss in primates, as rhythmic hind limb behavior and physiological responses could not be evoked in either chronic or acute spinal macaque monkeys (Edilberg et al. 1981). This observation was surprising since the supraspinal control of locomotion was reasonably similar in the cat and monkey. Since that time, there has been much experimentation in animals addressing this question with inconclusive results, and attempts at exciting CPG-like responses in spinal injured-human patients is still problematic (Dimitrijevic et al. 1998). Cases of so-called spinal stepping in neurologically complete human paraplegics is hard to confirm as occurring in complete isolation from any residual descending control. Curiously, in cases where stepping movements can be elicited in complete paraplegic humans, this happens in a waking state or state of near arousal, but usually not during sleep. This further supports the dominance of the brainstem in the control of human locomotion. The answer to the question of CPGs in humans may have been obvious for a long time: the most important anatomical location of something akin to a CPG in humans likely exists in the brainstem (Martin 1967) and not in the spinal cord as in quadrupeds. For an informative review of these issues, see Mori et al. (1996).

At the very least, the difficulty, indeed controversy, in revealing human CPGs analogous to animals tells even the casual reader of this literature that there exists significant differences in the control of purposeful locomotion between humans and other vertebrates. Even given the acknowledged inconsistencies in this literature, there are some optimistic rehabilitation researchers (Edgerton et al. 1992) who believe one may tap into hypothesized CPGs in the human to facilitate standing and walking after spinal cord injury, as normally occurs in four-legged animals (summarized by Wickelgren 1998; Edgerton et al. 1992; Illis 1995). Most proponents at least point out that a rehabilitation therapy aimed at generating locomotion by exciting CPG activity may more likely be meaningful for incomplete patients who retain significant white matter (Barbeau et al. 1998, 1999). This brings us full circle – to what degree would improved ambulation in neurologically incomplete patients be controlled by the brain or the spinal cord? This of course matters little to the patient who, through modern rehabilitation techniques, may stand and walk better than expected. However, these considerations matter greatly to the experimentalist studying walking behavior(s) in animals as a model for human paralysis. These two systems of purposeful locomotion are not analogous. As I tell lay groups and students, it is far easier for an engineer to build – or repair – a picnic table that remains upright on four legs – than one with two.

Methods that attempt to evaluate walking behavior after SCI in laboratory animals attempt to reconcile these daunting problems by a seemingly simple determination of whether the fore and hind limbs are coordinated during walking (Beatie et al. 1990; Cheng et al. 1997). This judgment is usually based on a subjective, or only partially quantitative, interpretation of locomotor movements, and usually without the benefit of kinesthesiological documentation. The return of stepping behavior after spinal injury in response to an experimental treatment elevates this state of confusion. One might reasonably suggest that functional neural transmission is re-established through the lesion in response to an experimental therapy (deemed not to occur in control animals) but not to the extent required to support truly coordinated ambulation.

5.1.1
The BBB Evaluation

In recent years a standardized behavioral analysis protocol has been developed by Ohio State University researchers Michael Beattie, Jackylin Bresnahan, and Michelle Basso (hence the adopted name, the BBB system, after the initials of its inventors), which is becoming widely used (Basso et al. 1996). Like other areas of medical research requiring complicated surgery and behavioral analysis, standardization of techniques is a worthy goal. Not knowing these individuals personally, we inquired into the technique and requested a reprint, and were surprised to receive a package of materials including sample score sheets, a VHS instructional video, even a question-and-answer text covering the most common areas of use and misuse of the method. Through a mutual friend, John Gruner, I learned that the Ohio State team provides this package to researchers, which makes their effort doubly worthwhile. Given the growing use of this tool for behavioral analysis, it deserves special comment here.

The BBB method is based upon a method of scoring hind limb load bearing, hind limb movement, and overall locomotor ability in paralyzed animals where 0 is the lowest score (completely paraplegic) and the highest score is 21 (a normal animal). The authors suggest means of prodding animals to attempt movement on a recommended surface and video taping their performance. Scoring is best achieved by blinded evaluation of these permanent records. As stated, I do not take seriously any claim of recovery from SCI based solely on locomotor behavior in quadrupeds. However, on balance, BBB scores that exceed the approximate median of 9/10 suggest performance likely based on restored conduction of nerve impulses through the lesion, a recovery producing coordination between hind and fore limbs. In practice, this is difficult to ascertain precisely at the breakpoint in the BBB scale below the median (8/9), but with animals scoring 11/12 points or higher, the task is easier and the interpretation less questionable. Scores below 8/9 lead us back into the swamp, even though they may be based on differing capabilities in limb movement between animals in the study groups. This is because movement of limbs in nonambulatory, even poorly ambulatory, animals is either based on local reflex activity or unknown. Differences in load bearing and uncoordinated stepping cannot be interpreted as being due to recovery of conduction through the lesion, which is the goal of any potential therapy for SCI. Let us explore this further with a bit of a digression from the laboratory to the clinic and back again.

In human or veterinary clinical medicine, injury or disease of the CNS is defined as being either an "upper motor neuron" or "lower motor neuron" syndrome. In the context of SCI, the former term refers to the local injury of the cord interfering with, or eliminating, neural communication between supraspinal motor centers and the motor neurons of the cord's gray matter that more often than not remain viable after injury. The latter term describes conditions that interfere with or eliminate neural communication between the motor neurons of the spinal cord and their target muscles. In the context of SCI, lower motor neuron sequelae can be due to the wholesale destruction of all motor neurons projecting axons to one or more extremities, trauma or disease of spinal roots or the PNS, and result in paralysis. Remember that cell death in the gray matter of typical spinal injuries (of approximately one vertebral segment in extent) will not denervate muscles of the limbs. Clinically, lower motor neuron signs occur most commonly in response to a variety of conditions producing ischemic injury to the entire lower spinal cord, for example, after clamping of arterial feeders to the spinal cord during emergency treatment and/or surgery or systemic trauma such as a burst aorta. In spinal-injured dogs, an insidious condition called ascending/descending myelomalacia can occur, resulting in a shift from upper motor neuron signs to lower motor neuron signs. This is due to a steady, progressive liquefaction of the cord over days to weeks, necessitating euthanasia. (Incidentally, this is likely a manifestation of extreme and unabated secondary injury processes in a naturally occurring clinical model.)

Clinical researchers should make every effort to exclude lower motor neuron animals (or people) from the study population since they do not possess the neural machinery to respond to a potential therapy aimed at restoring nerve impulse conduction through the spinal lesion. Lower motor neuron syndromes are diagnosed by the persistent dampening or lack of spinal reflexes (hyporeflexia or areflexia) and decreased muscle tone (Oliver and Mayhew 1983). In clinical trials using naturally spinal-injured dogs, we have even used the results of cystometry and urethral pressure profilometry, in addition to spinal reflex testing, to identify, and exclude, lower motor neuron dogs from the study population (Borgens et al. 1999). Upper motor neuron signs include normal to exaggerated spinal reflexes (hyperreflexia) and increased muscle tone. In people, such neurological testing is only informative after the transient period of spinal shock subsides since spinal reflexes are diminished or absent during this time (Tator 1995; Landy 1995). I do not know of any clear evidence for spinal shock in laboratory animal models of SCI. As mentioned, if there is any change in reflex movement of the limbs after SCI, they are usually exaggerated since the spinal injury interferes with or eliminates descending inhibition of spinal reflex circuits. The triggers for reflexive movement of limbs are many, varied, and many times unknown, not just limited to the investigator poking or prodding the animal's extremity. I have commonly observed spinal dogs begin pedaling movements of the legs when simply lifted to the examining table.

This brings us back to the BBB evaluation. It is hard to imagine how a standardized spinal injury to the thoracic spinal cord of an adult rat or guinea pig could produce lower motor neuron signs commonly observed in the clinic. All animal models of SCI useful to the researcher should thus show evidence of intact spinal reflexes, and these animals would be expected to exhibit movements in the lower limbs. From another point of view, this calls into question the meaning of such movements and the differences in them between animals with mean BBB scores of 8/9 or below. Are improvements in such scores representative of restored integrity of white matter and conduction through the spinal lesion? The best answer is that there is not an answer. Certainly claims of recovery of function after SCI (implying a positive effect of the treatment on the biology of the lesion) are unjustified based solely on this result. In what is called in the press an unscientific poll, I reviewed ten SCI reports using the BBB scoring system easily accessible to me, and did not find one study reporting mean improvements in any group of study animals in excess of 10/11. Most of the best average scores per group fell well below 10. All investigations claimed an enhanced recovery from SCI, or a recovery of function resulting from the experimental treatment. Only one report of the ten (McDonald et al. 1999) tempered this claim, declared in the title of the paper, with the following statement in the text: *"The BBB locomotor score differences between transplanted and control rats were not in the portion of the scale sensitive to forelimb-hindlimb coordination, so this study did not address whether functional connections improved across the lesion site"* (p 1411). What then, was the nature of the so-called recovery? These difficulties do not originate in the helpful BBB method. They arise from a failure of the investigators who use the method to properly understand or respect the limits of its interpretative power. Finally, variations of this evaluation tool are beginning to show up in the literature: all that I have studied fall short of the original. Some investigators attempt to compress the 0–21 scale of the BBB method into a 0–6 or 0–5 scale. This is unacceptable because, in these cases, the scores were not weighted properly relative to coordinated stepping as attempted in the original method. For example, in one case (Vacanti et al. 2001) all BBB scores between 13 and 21 were compressed into the single highest grade achievable (6), the lowest score remained 0 (as in the BBB method), while a score of 1 combined BBB scores of 1 and 2. All of the individual grades from 0–4 represented nonambulatory animals, while 5 and 6 represented ambulatory ones – serving to artificially inflate the performance scores of the worst responders.

Overall, the presence and expression of hindlimb reflexes both complicate and confuse claims of "behavioral" recovery in much of this literature. Moreover, there are clear *species* differences in the reflex response to mechanical stimulation. For a clear example refer to a discussion of the difference in the flexor withdrawal reflex in guinea pigs and rats in Gruner et al. (1996; p 98). Rats may be generally hyporeflexive normally – however this "dampened" state should be unmasked by spinal cord injury. Clear evidence of *hyperactive* reflex responses in spinal animals is everywhere – when one looks for it. Friedman et al. (2000) used the *reduction* in hyperflexia of the tail in spinal cats as a functional indicator of the success of *re-establishing descending* inhibition after fetal cell transplants. Careful evaluation of such issues is curiously absent from most SCI behavioral testing – which plods along with prompted motor functions in rats (usually) and scoring all of the control animals as "zeros".

5.1.2
Novel Behavioral Indices of White Matter Integrity

Some scientists have realized the possibilities inherent in using functional indexes for behavioral recovery in laboratory animals other than walking and stepping. One interesting individual was the creative spinal cord scholar, the late Michael Goldberger of the University of Pennsylvania. He clearly pointed out the benefits of using various proprioceptive (particularly tactile) placing behaviors of the hind limbs in laboratory animals. Some of these behaviors can easily be documented and quantified and some are based on partially identified neural circuitry, with a behavioral expression that can be permanently abolished by spinal injury (Goldberger 1980; see also Bregman et al. 1994).

In the early 1980s I became increasingly frustrated with the considerable unknowns in evaluating walking in spinal rodents, and the propensity for false-positives when evaluating recovery from spinal injury in guinea pigs and rats. In response to this frustration, our laboratory adopted another type of long tract reflex, called the cutaneus trunci muscle reflex (CTM) as a tool to evaluate behavioral recovery in rats and guinea pigs. The CTM reflex (also called the panniculus reflex by veterinarians) was first explored systematically by Jack Diamond's group at McMaster University in the adult rat (Theriault and Diamond 1988a, b). Andrew Blight and I worked out this neural circuit in the guinea pig and a means to quantify the behavior (Blight et al. 1990) (Fig. 10). We have employed this model for over 15 years. The behavior is a reflexive contraction of the skin of the back, sometimes appearing as a

--▶

Fig. 10. The cutaneous trunci muscle (*CTM*) reflex as a behavioral index for spinal cord injury. On the *left side* of the guinea pig, the afferent and efferent pathways of the CTM reflex are diagrammed. Nociceptive receptors in the skin project sensory afferents (*green*) into the spinal cord via the dorsal cutaneous nerves (*DCNs*). DCNs are segmentally organized, are arranged roughly parallel to each other, are perpendicular to the spinal cord, and project into the spinal cord as a component of the dorsal roots. The ascending CTM afferents project up the spinal cord as a tract. The CTM tract is located just lateral to the spinothalamic tract in the ventral funiculus on both right and left sides. Very few relays make up the ascending tract, which projects onto a pool of motor neurons (*red*) located at the cervical/thoracic junction. These in turn project efferent motor fibers (*blue*) back to the cutaneus trunci muscle of the skin via the lateral thoracic branch of the brachial plexus. A neural connection between left and right motor neuron pools does not exist, though there is minor contralateral innervation within the spinal cord's ascending CTM projections (not shown). On the right side of the guinea pig's spinal cord (*light yellow*), a spinal injury (a large gap for illustrative purposes) interrupts the ascending CTM tract on only that side. Note that this produces a region of back skin that no longer responds to tactile stimulation (it is areflexic). This region of areflexia is ipsilateral and below the level of this right lateral hemisection of the spinal cord. Note that the CTM reflex ipsilateral and above, and contralateral to, the injury is not affected. A full-width injury compromising both CTM tracts would eliminate skin responsiveness on both sides of the animal below the lesion. The back skin rostral to the injury would be unaffected by this spinal cord injury. This is shown in the video reconstructions *below*. From *left to right* – the *first picture* shows an intact CTM receptive field *outlined in green*. Tactile probing within this area produced twitching of the back skin, and outside of this region, stimulation did not produce CTM skin contractions. This series of light tactile stimulations of the skin of a sedated animal is videotaped from above and the drawings

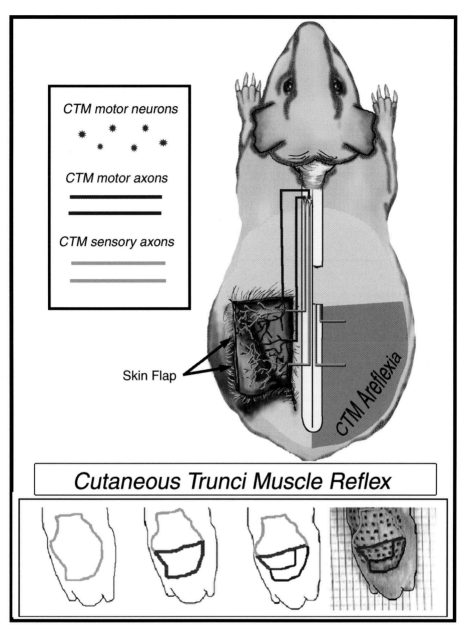

CTM motor neurons

CTM motor axons

CTM sensory axons

Skin Flap

CTM Areflexia

Cutaneous Trunci Muscle Reflex

reconstructed by computer. The *second picture* shows the results of a full-width spinal cord compression injury. The region *outlined in red* is the region of areflexia – that is – the lower half of the CTM receptive field that no longer responds to tactile stimulation. The *third drawing* reveals a region of CTM recovery *outlined in blue*. Within this region, CTM responsiveness has returned. The *last image* is a frame from the videotape showing the grid of dots tattooed on the animals shaved back. This grid is useful for further quantification of the CTM reflex, combined with the outlines drawn on the animal's back with markers during CTM testing

rippling in response to light tactile stimulation. Anyone who has watched horses grazing on a hot summer's day usually remembers the strong corrugated rippling of the skin of the back and flank, the swishing of the tail, when the horse was pestered by flies. That strong rhythmic contraction of skin is the behavioral expression of the CTM reflex. The important points below demonstrate its usefulness to the SCI investigator.

1. Unlike walking behavior, the anatomy of the complete sensory and motor circuitry of the CTM reflex, both in the CNS and PNS, has been identified (Blight et al. 1990; Thierault and Diamond 1988) (Fig. 10). This known architecture provides the investigator additional means to directly test the anatomical basis of functional recovery of the CTM (refer to Fig. 10 in Borgens et al. 1990).
2. The CTM behavior is easy to illicit through light tactile stimulation of the back skin (with a probe or fine bristle brush) and easy to document in the sedate or quiet animal using real-time video recording. The complex behavior of skin contractions can be quantified; the velocity, vector, and latency of skin movement in response to stimulation can be determined, as well as the unit area of both CTM sensitive skin and the region of areflexia caused by the spinal cord injury (see Blight et al. 1990; Borgens et al. 2002). Severing or crushing the CTM tracts within the cord results in a region of the receptive field that no longer responds to tactile stimulation (the region of areflexia) (Fig. 10). This areflexia is produced below the level of injury and ipsilateral to it. Compensatory cutaneous sprouting into this region of back skin from adjacent functional skin does not occur because the region of areflexic skin is not denervated. The peripheral circuitry is completely intact and the behavioral deficit is due to a central lesion.
3. The functional characteristics of the CTM for an individual animal can be documented prior to injury and any recovery of function can then be compared to this normal pattern.
4. The ascending CTM tract is located lateral to the spinothalamic tract in the ventral funiculus of the cord on both sides of the midline. Following transection of the CTM tract on one or both sides, the CTM reflex is lost below the level of the injury for the life of the animal (Borgens et al. 1987, 1990, 1993; Blight et al. 1990). We have never observed a spontaneous recovery of the CTM reflex in over 120 animals (in published reports) subsequent to confirmed transection of the CTM tract (refer to Borgens et al. 1987, 1990; Metcalf et al. 1993). Moreover, the frequency of spontaneous recovery subsequent to a standardized compression injury to the cord is low – usually less than 20% of the control population. I have admitted that the CTM reflex is not, in itself, relevant to human medicine – as humans do not have a CTM reflex. Clinical recovery of function is best evaluated in a clinical model, such as naturally injured canines as discussed in Chap. 14, "Naturally Occurring Spinal Injury in the Dog as a Model for Humans" (Borgens 1992). The CTM reflex, however, provides a clear answer to the question of whether this experimental therapy can reverse or improve functional loss that would not otherwise occur in the control animals in laboratory investigations.

5.2
Injuring the Cord and Probing Its Anatomy

In addition to concerns over behavioral evaluation, numerous and varied techniques have been offered to induce injury to the exposed spinal cord in laboratory animals. In contrast to the human injury, all modern laboratory injuries are made to the dorsal aspect of surgically exposed spinal cords of anesthetized animals. This is inconsistent with clinical injuries where the injuries are usually anterior (ventral), and the neuroprotective attributes of anesthesia are not a complicating factor (Salzman et al. 1990). The direct mechanical injury is to the trunk of the body or neck, a so-called closed injury.

In animal models of SCI, constant impact (usually standardized weight drop techniques; Allen 1911; Somerson and Stokes 1987), constant compression of the spinal cord using specially fabricated clips (Rivlin and Tator 1978) or forceps (Blight 1991) and partial or complete transection of the spinal cord (Borgens et al. 1986a) have all been employed and contrasted. With the exception of the latter technique, the goals have been to reduce the variability in the characteristics of the lesion between animals and to produce a central hemorrhagic injury somewhat typical of clinical injury in humans. Transection, on the other hand, has been used almost exclusively in recent years to study axonal regeneration in the spinal cord. In regeneration studies it is important to know axons were actually severed, and that intracellular labels are not marking crushed but intact fibers remaining within the lesion (see Chap. 6, Sect. 6.1.1, "Marking the Lesion").

Though we cannot label and trace identified axons in the mammalian cord as we can in simply organized vertebrates such as the ammocoete lamprey, one can use intracellular labels to mark identified long tracts or columns of axons in the white matter. The modern use of intracellular labels, such as horseradish peroxidase and various fluorescently decorated dextrans, has improved our powers of evaluation over the historical use of silver impregnation techniques. Intracellular labels can be introduced to the spinal cord tissue by injection; they are imbibed by the injured axons at the injection site and moved along the length of axons by anterograde and retrograde transport. Techniques examining anterograde transport of dyes to the axon terminal and retrograde transport – to mark the cell body – are commonly used to evaluate the anatomy of the injury. However, there are many pitfalls. In any spinal lesion where the superficial investments of the cord are compromised, normally regenerating axons of the PNS can gain access to spinal cord parenchyma (Ramón y Cajal 1928; Barnes and Worrall 1968; Beattie et al. 1997). These regenerating axons can originate from nearby spinal roots that may have been compromised by the surgery as well. One can reduce or eliminate the possibility of confusing these axons with CNS axons by labeling both the cord's long tracts and spinal roots near the lesion with separate markers or by simply injecting a few microliters of one marker into select white matter tracts over two vertebral segments from the lesion (Borgens and Bohnert 1997). An alternate route of dye uptake by axons peripheral to the cord is highly unlikely using this method and appropriate controls. Recently, a unique approach has been used to specifically address these difficulties. As discussed previously, mice were genetically engineered to express green fluorescence protein (GFP) in their cells. Thus, transplanted GFP neurons and their regenerating processes stood out dramatically against the background tissues of the host rats (Davies et al. 1999).

It is important to trace the lengths of axons within the white matter tracts and the lesion longitudinally, so their origin and terminals can be confirmed. Counting of axons contained within cross sections on the other side of the injury from where the label was introduced, is insufficient data on which to base claims of axonal regeneration. The longitudinal camera lucida (usually composite) drawings showing the spotty presence of labeling on the other side of the lesion from where an anterograde marker was applied is also insufficient grounds to claim axonal regeneration. This is because the source of these axons cannot be precisely verified and are unaccompanied by anatomical documentation of their terminal endings across the plane of transection. This is especially true when studying the anatomy of compression injuries of the cord where it is very difficult to distinguish damaged but surviving axons from regenerating ones. Personally, I do not take seriously any claim of axonal regeneration that uses these techniques even if there are significantly increased numbers of labeled axons in response to the experimental treatment. Perhaps the experimental treatment increased axonal sparing (in compression lesions) but did not facilitate regenerative growth. Perhaps the attempted transection was incomplete, which can occur sometimes in even experienced laboratories. Alternately or additionally, perhaps the experimental treatment increased collateral sprouting from intact fibers surviving the crush injury (discussed in Chap. 7, Sect. 7.3, "Regeneration") or the branching of such collaterals.

6 Axonal Regeneration

Most scholars agree that the first scientist to clearly describe axonal regeneration (as we now know it) was the Englishman William Cumberland Cruikshank about the time of the signing of the American Declaration of Independence in 1776 (Ochs 1977). The search for a practical means to regenerate CNS axons has become the Holy Grail for the students of CNS injury. This requires not only a means to induce more robust powers of growth in surviving proximal segments of axons, but to provide directional cues to them during regeneration as well. Santiago Ramón y Cajal (1928) explained what experimental neurology must do to realize this dream: (The neurologist) *"must give to the sprouts, by means of adequate alimentation, a vigorous capacity for growth; and place in front of the disoriented nerve cones and in the thickness of the tracts of the white matter and neuronic foci specific orienting substances"* (Ramón y Cajal 1928, p 738).

Only a few years ago, Professor Anders Björklund of the University of Lund in Sweden, stated this same opinion in nearly identical terms: *"The big challenge in spinal cord regeneration research is to find ways to stimulate axonal regrowth, and to modify the properties of axonal growth trajectory in the damaged cord, in order to reestablish enough functional supraspinal connections with isolated spinal cord segments"* (Björklund 1994, p 112–113).

Many experimental approaches make use of existing neural machinery surviving the insult, or attempt to rescue it from degeneration (see Chap. 7, "Treatment Possibilities of the New Biology"). A regeneration therapy is intended to create new neural circuits. Recall the earlier discussion that these new connections do not need to be appropriate connections. Ramón y Cajal also understood that it was not necessary to initiate axonal regeneration in fibers that are unable to extend themselves. It is more an issue to facilitate the abortive regeneration that spontaneously begins in severed CNS tracts – but is vitiated prematurely. *"It cannot be denied, therefore, that the central axons have the property of producing new fibers, and what has to be explained is why, once the reconstructive movement is initiated, the nerve sprouts lose their energy and suspend their growth"* (Ramón y Cajal 1928, p 745).

The issue of collateral sprouting deserves special mention. It is acknowledged that axonal regeneration is the ability to extend the tip of the proximal segment of a severed axon, succinctly stated by Kiernan. *"It must be emphasized that this sequence of events, known as axonal regeneration, is one in which cells are replacing their amputated cytoplasmic processes"* (Kiernan 1979, p 156).

Moreover, it is this capability, characteristic of myelinated axons, that is dramatically reduced in the mammalian CNS.

6.1
Collateral Sprouting

Collateral sprouting, also called reactive reinnervation, is a phenomenon where neurons increase their terminal fields by the sometimes extensive growth of new fibers (a.k.a. sprouts). The formation of sprouts from an axotomized nerve fiber occurs proximal to the tip of the amputated fiber. Growth from the tip of the proximal segment is axonal regeneration. Sprouting from the membrane quite proximal to the tip is referred to as compensatory sprouting, as distinct from collateral sprouting, which occurs in intact axons, which may be nearby (Goldberger et al. 1993). The capacity to form sprouts throughout the life of the mammal in the brain and in the spinal cord is an expression of plasticity, the regulative ability of neural circuits to maintain and shape themselves in response to changing conditions such as injury or disease. Both collateral and compensatory sprouting can occur regularly and extensively in the adult mammal in response to various and many different stimuli. Even in Alzheimer's disease, a condition associated with the aged, sprouting not only occurs in and around the b-amyloid protein plaques, but also may actually contribute to their formation (Cotman et al. 1993). They write: "These findings support the hypothesis that the aged brain is capable of reactive synaptogenesis" (Cotman et al. 1993, p 226). Collateral and compensatory sprouting occurs most readily in the younger animal, particularly in the postnatal period where the brain is still developing its circuitry.

The upside of these facts, also described and discussed by Ramón y Cajal, is that they offer evidence that regenerative growth and synaptogenesis can be expected to be facilitated in the CNS of the adult mammal. There is no downside, except for the experimentalist who does not expend the effort to prove what is claimed to be CNS axonal regeneration is not in fact a sprouting phenomenon. One phenomenon is recalcitrant in the CNS of the adult mammal, the other can occur with facility. I have been impressed with how many regeneration and transplantation studies are carried out in very young rats, 2–5 weeks old. This is the first clue for the critical reader to look more closely at the both the claim of axonal regeneration and the documentation of it.

Sprouting can be regulated or initiated by many sorts of factors such as repeated transections, the natural or experimental liberation of neurotrophic factors, even the animal's state of health. In most cases, the very experimental variable the investigator believes should produce axonal regeneration is likely to facilitate sprouting as well, and it is incumbent on the scientist to delineate these possibilities.

6.1.1
Marking the Lesion

A marker device or some other implementation should be used to clearly determine the original plane of the transection in studies of spinal cord axon regeneration. Spinal lesions can be quite extended in surface area within the vertebral segment of cord that is damaged. Cut axons die back like a cigarette burning back in the ashtray (Fig. 11). Significant retrograde degeneration (dieback) of severed axons is typical of most axons, and this distance is highly variable. The tips of the proximal segments

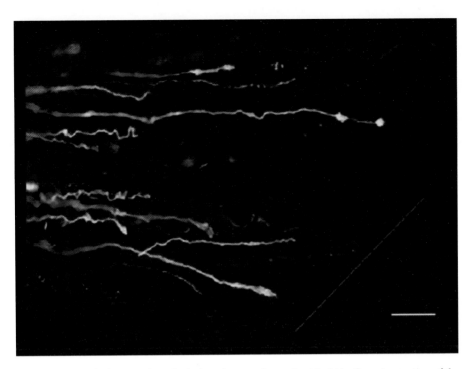

Fig. 11. Retrograde degeneration of spinal cord axons. Approximately 14 h after a transection of the spinal cord (*hatched line*), axons have both pulled back, or died back, from the cut edge. The swollen tips (degeneration clubs) probably reveal axons that are undergoing retrograde degeneration. Some coiled axons are also seen in all preparations such as this, suggesting a physical springing back from the injury. Spinal cords are quite elastic, requiring a degree of pliability to conform with movements of the body. Thus, axons are elastic as well and can pop backwards from the plane of an injury when severed. The scale bar is approximately 40 μm

of severed axons must regenerate back to the plane of transection if they are to cross it. If axons indeed die back over a centimeter (not uncommon) and then regenerate half of this distance (reasonably impressive), how would the investigator know this, or even document this regeneration, if the exact plane of transection is either lost or obscured within the disorganized, sometimes extensive scar tissue formed during the weeks and months after surgery? Sometimes, investigators interpret the swollen terminals of anterograde-filled proximal segments as regenerating. This practice is also fraught with difficulty since the swollen ends of degenerating proximal segments (called end bulbs or clubs) can appear remarkably similar to that of growth cones when observed in whole mounts of cleared spinal cord tissues (see Borgens et al. 1986a). Though the need for establishing the plane of transection to enable credible documentation of regeneration has been discussed for over 30 years (see Foerster 1982; Borgens et al. 1986a), the use of indwelling markers to establish this plane is rarely employed. Sometimes it has been claimed that they are, though the reader was not provided documentation of their use (Schnell and Schwab 1990). This does not then do much to support the claim of axonal elongation past the level of transection.

Of course the foregoing discussion applies to tracing axonal trajectories through the parenchyma of the spinal cord. These considerations apply less to experiments where alternate pathways for axonal regeneration are provided such as peripheral nerve bridges spanning the lesion (David and Aguayo 1981) or hollow polymeric tubes into which axons may be coaxed to regenerate (Borgens 1999). These techniques provide unambiguous proof of axonal regeneration, though the origin of the fibers entering and/or traversing the foreign pathways must still be properly established as being of CNS or PNS origin. This can be accomplished by retrograde labeling of the cell bodies or fiber tracts giving rise to fibers labeled within the artificial pathway. Finally, special histochemistry is usually required to reveal the small diameter (≤ 1 μm) cholinergic and adrenergic fibers of the spinal cord. These naturally regenerate after spinal cord damage (Björklund and Stenevi 1972; Björklund et al. 1971, 1973) and one should always be mindful of this when evaluating the anatomy of experimentally treated spinal cords for evidence of axonal regeneration. Small labeled fibers coursing along with newly formed capillaries would be especially suspicious.

It would surprise the reader to know that most well-accepted claims of axonal regeneration within the spinal cord of mammals in the modern literature do not employ such safeguards or utilize more rigorous techniques to properly document their claims – and are thus suspect.

6.2
A Neuron's Journey: Integrating Guidance Cues

I have been discussing the formation of new growth in nerve processes. The student investigator must understand the means by which nerve fibers are thought to find their targets during development – particularly when considering potential therapies that may initiate the extension of nerve fibers, and their guidance, in the adult.

The amount and complexity of cell guidance during development and regeneration is nearly unfathomable. An attempt to decipher this code we must – if we are to understand not only our own beginnings, but also gain mastery over disease and injury.

This text centers on injury to the CNS, particularly the spinal cord, so I will briefly discuss tropic and trophic cues relative to neurons, though much of this discussion applies to many types of cells. The neuron is special, however. Not only do neurons take up, or relocate to, special locations within the developing nervous system as they are born, but their growing processes must navigate an extraordinarily complex terrain. This terrain is loaded with both guiding and confusing factors, but still the advancing fibers must make connections with appropriate targets at appropriate times. Sometimes this recognition and target acquisition is highly specific, while an alternative strategy is to make thousands of new connections, letting degenerative processes and cell death prune and shape the neural circuit to its final form (Cowan et al. 1984). These tasks are made even more complicated since the entire environment surrounding cells groping their way through this maze is expanding in size and complexity as well.

It has been known for over 100 years that the most important components of the map for directed guidance cues are extrinsic ones – those provided by the environment. The earliest observations of contact guidance by the best of our scientific fore-fathers, Santiago Ramón y Cajal and Ross Harrison, for example, revealed that growing nerve processes make choices depending on the surfaces they come into contact with. It is clear that the entire cell and its innards of organelles and transport machinery are involved in making this choice, though the initial sensor is likely the filopodia of the growth cone. Amoeboid filopodia extend and retract, extend and retract – constantly sampling the local and long-distance cues provided by the roads ahead. The nerve cell must continuously sample and interpret this changing topography as well as cues provided in its aqueous environment. Commonly, filopodia are most numerous and active on the side of the growth cone favoring a turn in this direction. It is also believed that the turn itself is a biomechanical event, where tensional forces (push or pull) exerted through actin/myosin-type microfilaments reshape the architecture of the fiber terminal (Letourneau et al. 1987, 1991; Bray 1987). These changes in the anatomy of the growth cone are transduced by a dizzying array of interactions between the cytoskeleton, membrane spanning proteins that are attached to it, the specific influence on these proteins by molecular cues in the microenvironment, and the gating of ions (principally Ca^{++}) across the membrane (Fig. 12).

Having said all this, it is likely that filopodia exert a permissive influence on directed growth of the nerve fiber, and not an instructive one, since growth cones deprived of filopodia (e.g., by treatment with cytochalasin D) can, under experimental conditions, still respond to orientation cues (see McCaig 1989; Marsh and Letourneau 1984). However, like the growth cone, we will stay largely on track here and hold digressions to a minimum, important as they may be. Finally, nerves elongate by the addition of new membrane at the base of the cone – so perhaps a rate-limiting step in nerve growth is the anterograde movement of membrane precursors by axoplasmic transport (principally the slow transport mechanisms).

6.2.1
Roadways

Before exploring the interactions of universally recognized guidance cues with extracellular electric fields, it should be remembered, if not emphasized, that in nature many such factors are simultaneously presented to the advancing growth cone. There is little evidence to suggest that individual navigational cues are temporally and spatially arranged for the advancing nerve process to read. This would reduce complex cellular navigation to simple recognition of a hierarchy. Rather, nerve cells must be able to integrate these many and variable cues in order to act on them. Most developmentalists know this; however, the foundations of this science have been largely based on studying the action of one guidance cue in isolation from the others, which sometimes unfortunately entrains our thinking.

There are four general categories of extrinsic factors that serve as cues for the navigation of growing and regenerating nerve processes. My number 1 – and the least appreciated by cell biologists – is an endogenous extracellular DC voltage gradient (Chapt. 8, "Biologically Produced Electrical Fields: Physiology Spoken Here", and Chap. 12, "Recovery of the CTM Reflex in Spinal Injured Guinea Pigs After Exposure to Applied Extracellular Voltages"). The others are:

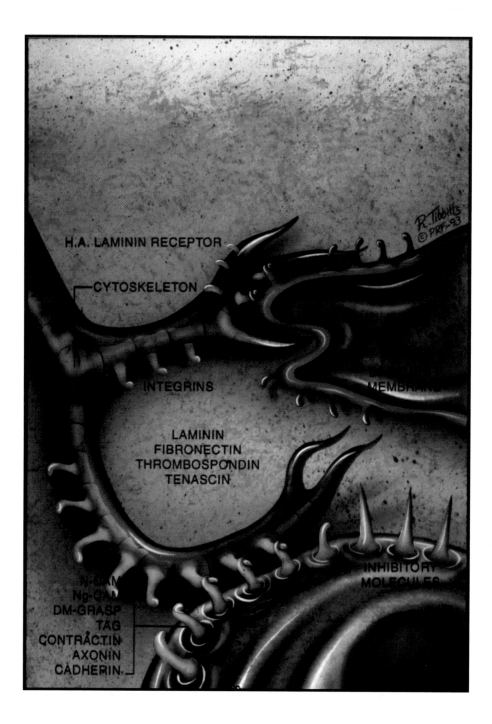

2. Specific chemical mediators, which may be bound or soluble: the so-called growth factors such as nerve growth factor (NGF), brain-derived neural growth factor (BDNF), neurotrophins (NT) 3–5, as well as neurotransmitter substances such as acetyl choline (ACh) and glutamate released into the extracellular space, which have more recently been discovered to play this role as well.
3. Gradients of adhesivity or repulsion – characteristic of specific extracellular matrix substrates such as laminin, fibronectin, tenascin, collagen, or specific molecules inserted in the membranes of cells such as neuronal cell adhesion molecules (NCAMs) or inhibitory molecules such as some proteoglycans, and N250 and N35 based on introductory statements in the previous paragraph.
4. Surface characteristics of the topography (as opposed to its chemical characteristics).

Starting with the last point, there are many landmark observations in biology of directed cell growth following preformed pathways: the radial glia scaffolding providing a template for the navigation of developing brain neurons championed by Pasco Rakic; the substrate slings of tissue in developing brain elaborated more recently by Jerry Silver; the bands of Bungner providing growth surfaces for regeneration as discussed by Santiago Ramón y Cajal; and the classic observations of Marcus Singer, Ruth Nordlander, and Margaret Egar of glial channels forming out of scar tissue in transected salamander spinal cord for regenerating axons to subsequently follow. These three pioneers called functional spinal cord regeneration through such channels the blueprint hypothesis (Singer et al. 1979). It is possible that surface irregularities are just as important as the chemical composition and characteristics of the organic substrate in controlling cell movements – easily demonstrated by neurons guiding on a scratch in the bottom of the culture dish. This feature of contact guidance has been largely ignored until recently, which is why I will expand on this issue first.

Recent advancements in nanofabrication techniques have allowed a deeper probing of this issue (for examples see Nagata et al. 1993; Rajnicek et al. 1997). The latter investigators used a directed electron beam lithography process to directly write in-

---

Fig. 12. Signposts and roadways during cell movement. This drawing shows some of the major factors governing the course of directed cell movement. In the *blue* cell process at the *bottom*, various cell adhesion molecules spanning the membrane are named, all of which have an affinity for corresponding molecules (integrins) protruding from the branching red process. Note that these membrane-spanning molecules are usually connected with the cytoskeleton of the cell as drawn. The tip of the branched *red* process at the *bottom* is pulling away from a membrane-bound putative inhibitory molecule (such as myelin-associated protein or rTAPA) as discussed in the text. The surface that these cells reside on (*in yellow gold*) is named for the common extracellular matrix molecules (ECMs), each with different levels of adhesiveness for the various and different cells that may contact them. As shown in the branching *red* nerve process at the *top*, there are specialized receptors for such ECM molecules. The roadway (as described in the text) is the extracellular matrix, deposited by other types of cells not shown, though some cells deposit their own "asphalt" in advance of their movements. The ECM provides more of a continuous signaling to motile cells. The interactions between CAMs and integrins are more discontinuous, depending on the types of cells that interact; thus these are by analogy the signposts in the cell's journey

credibly precise grooves in fused quartz (with standardized depths as little as 14 nm). They posed various questions to both embryonic *Xenopus* spinal neurons and rat hippocampal neurons cultured on flat quartz surfaces, comparing the choices growing fibers were forced to make when encountering nano-grooves of precisely varying dimensions. Mammalian hippocampal neurons favored wide (4 µm) and deep (500–1,000 nm) channels for maximum parallel contact guidance. In narrow (1 µm) and shallow (130 nm) grooves, the same neurons projected axons perpendicular to the grooves. Frog neurons behaved completely differently. Their neurites demonstrated typical parallel contact guidance with grooves that was very narrow *and* very shallow (1 µm×130 nm). They guided similarly on grooves of increasing widths and depths. On a more subtle level, grooves even affected the position on the cell body where neurites would emerge. *Xenopus* neurites emerged uniformly on the surface of somas grown on a quartz surfaces without grooves and those with shallow grooves (≤14 nm deep). If the depth of the grooves was more than doubled (to 36 nm) most neurites emerged on the side of the cell body parallel with the grooves. The responses by hippocampal neurons were more complicated and seemed to be determined by the kind of neurite growing out of the soma – be it axon or dendrite. Axons extended from the side of the cell body perpendicular to grooves and dendrites parallel to it. Finally, the rates of nerve growth were markedly enhanced when fibers were growing in a preferred direction determined by the characteristics of the groove (Rajnicek et al. 1997).

6.2.2
Signposts

While the topographic character of contact guidance is receiving more attention, the types of extracellular matrix molecules (ECM) have always been an important part of the lexicon of nerve growth and guidance. Molecular signaling to the advancing growth cone can be thought of as being both continuous and discontinuous in situ. Continuous signaling is provided by the expanses of ECM such as the ubiquitous matrix components laminin, fibronectin, and collagen, to name only a few. Where pathways in the embryo exist with relative higher compositions of these compounds, growth along these surfaces is likely. These paths are expressed as gradients in ECMs; they reduce or eliminate nonspecific wandering by growing processes when a favorable terrain is located, and create true fasciculation pathways – especially if adhesive pathways are bounded by repellent ECMs. Adhesivity involves many factors such as the surface area of contact between the motile lamellipodia or filopodia, regional differences in the selective gating of Ca^{++} into the filopodia (thought to occur at regions of membrane extension), and signal transduction by another type of transmembrane chemical component, the integrins. These membrane-spanning moieties are believed to connect with cytoskeletal proteins, the contractile and transport machinery of the cell (Fig. 12).

Intimate localizations occur between integrins and most of the family of microfilaments and tubulins found in the axons and growth cones such as actin, vinculin, and valine. There are also molecules inserted within the membranes of the cells themselves (as opposed to secretion products) that can provide discontinuous signaling. These molecules can be both attractive or repellent to advancing growth cones (inhibitory ones, such a myelin-associated proteins, are discussed in Chap. 3, Sect. 3.1, "Inhibitory Molecules"). Cell adhesion molecules (CAMS), including a family common to neurons (NCAMS) and cadherins, are other examples. This signaling is discontinuous because pathway selection depends on the cell type encountered by growth cones during their journey. Loosely speaking, ECM is the asphalt and concrete of the roadway, while CAMS are the highway signs. As mentioned, mechanical forces associated with the contractile proteins and filaments within the growth cone help shape its architecture, so it is comforting to know that the cytoskeletal machinery of the cell is dynamically, yet still mechanically, linked to CAMS and ECMs by specialized transmembrane proteins (these complex issues are well organized and well explained in the informative review by Bixby and Harris 1991) (Fig. 12). The very change in growth cone shape, however, provides feedback to this molecule recognition system through the physiological properties of the membrane.

There are specialized ion channels that respond to changes in the physical characteristics of the membrane, the best studied being so-called stretch-activated potassium channels, which secondarily influence the gating of Ca^{++} through voltage gated channels, and therefore, local intracellular concentrations of calcium. These intracellular Ca^{++} fluctuations within the physiological range provide feedback to regulate cytoarchitecture. There is little dispute concerning this fact; however, there are differing views over the specific role of local gating of Ca^{++} into the growth cone (Palmer et al. 1997). My interpretation of this literature favors the notion that localized entry of Ca^{++} indeed predetermines growth cone orientation. This is a long-held bias, however, ever since observing vibrating electrode measurement of Ca^{++} currents traversing the presumptive rhizoid region of fucus eggs (Jaffe and Nuccitelli 1977) and entering the tip of extending pseudopods in giant amoeba (Nuccitelli et al. 1977) as a student in Lionel Jaffe's laboratory 30 years ago. Clearly, however, Ca^{++} entry within the physiological range favors an increase in the adhesiveness of the membrane to the substrate (Gunderson and Barrett 1980; Cohan et al. 1987). This does not occur in only filopodia, and may help explain the continued, albeit it weak, capability of a neurite to read substrate cues sans filopodia subsequent to cytochalasin treatment (McCaig 1989).

6.2.3
Growth Factors

Soluble factors, particularly the growth factors, a subfamily of cytokines, have been extensively researched for over 40 years. The characterization of nerve growth factor (NGF) by Rita Levi-Montalcini and the fortuitous discovery that the submandibular gland of male mice is rich with NGF was largely responsible for fast early strides in understanding neurotrophic factors. One could argue that this one event, in addition to the Watson and Crick paper in *Nature*, triggered the modern fascination with the biochemistry of development and genetics. In a classic 1960 paper, Stanley Cohen not only described how to purify NGF, but also revealed the destruction of the peripheral sympathetic system of neonates following injections of an anti-NGF antibody.

Peripheral sympathetic neurons have long been understood to respond most vigorously to NGF, though trophic support of sensory neurons and central cholinergic neurons has also been established. Here I am discussing the trophic support of neurons, that is, nourished and kept viable by trophic factors, Another example is BDNF. Though this factor is relatively low in abundance compared to NGF, there is considerable overlap in both of their abilities to support neuronal viability and to prevent experimentally induced cell death in vivo. (For reviews of the foundations of this modern science, see Levi-Montalcini and Angeletti 1968; Levi-Montalcini 1987; Barde 1989.) Trophic factors can usually induce tropic response in their specific class of responding neurons, that is, they can induce turning behavior and overall influence the directed growth of neuronal processes. I wish I had a nickel for every reviewer who chided my spelling for using the term "tropic factor." Trophic and tropic influences – or responses – are not the same. Nerve tropisms, or turning behaviors, are widely observed by producing a gradient of a soluble factor within the culture chamber by delivering it through a pipette and observing that neurites orient and track up this gradient to sometimes enter the pipette tip. The turning behavior of growth cones into the gradient has been enough to classically emphasize the neurotropic properties of NGF, and more recently ACh (Zheng et al. 1994), BDNF, netrin 1, NT-3, and glutamate (Zheng et al. 1996; Song et al. 1997; and Ming et al. 1997). I have never quite understood the reluctance of neurobiologists to as easily accept the fact that an imposed voltage gradient is as potent a neurotropic factor as these molecules since exactly the same experiment can be performed with exactly the same result. When one uses a micropipette as a cathode to produce a similar gradient, but in voltage, both the results and the experiments are exactly analogous.

In the context of spinal cord injury, trophic support of injured neurons in the gray matter is likely useful, but more important is the tropic effects of growth factors in addition to their ability to stimulate fiber outgrowth and branching. The messenger RNAs for a variety of neurotrophic factors have been found in spinal cord, including NGF, BDNF, the neurotropins (NT) 3–5, while in brain injury, these, as well as the cytokines FGFs, transforming growth factor (TGF-β) and CNTF, are expressed. The neuron's responses to these chemicals are mediated by specific receptors that can be characterized as having a high or low affinity for an individual neurotrophic factor or family. Thus, there are low-affinity NGF receptors and more specific high-affinity receptors (such as trkB and C). In general, many of the receptors continue to be expressed on neuronal surfaces through the life of the animal, while the concentrations of the neurotrophic factors are down-regulated late in postnatal development and/or soon after birth. This is reversible, obviously, with increased production of neurotrophic substances after injury by a host of cells, including nonneuronal cells such as fibroblasts, macrophages, and Schwann cells.

7 Treatment Possibilities of the New Biology

I sometimes describe the possible treatments for spinal injury in terms of the three Rs: restoration, repair, and regeneration of the nervous system. There is less overlap in these three categories than one would think.

7.1
Restoration

The concept of restoration involves a means of utilizing some of the anatomically spared nervous tissue remaining in the spinal cord after injury. Recall that the clinical injury primarily originates in the central regions of the spinal cord (gray matter) and spreads centrifugally. Cords progressively die from the inside out after mechanical damage (Fig. 4). In a neurologically complete injury – where there is no sensory or motor function preserved below the level of the injury – there is usually still a variable rim of spared white matter. This region of preservation extends for a variable distance beneath the pial surface. This anatomically intact rind of axons is, of course, not functional in neurologically complete injuries. Restoring it to function embodies the goal of the first R. Since these fibers do not support the conduction of nerve impulses through the lesion, the loss of behavioral function associated with them would be similar in consequence to a complete transection of the cord, a rare event in human spinal cord accidents. This failure in conductance is thought to be related to a focal demyelination of these axons, ionic derangement between the intracellular and extracellular compartments produced by the mechanical injury, and perhaps even autoimmune-mediated destruction of ion channels required for the initiation of action potentials.

7.1.1
Reversing the Physiological Conduction Block

Since establishment of the membrane potential of the axolemma is dominated by the Nernst potential for K^+, the unregulated intracellular loss of K^+ as it moves down its electrochemical gradient out of the damaged membrane leads to an increase in the K^+ concentration of the extracellular microenvironment. This increase in extracellular potassium facilitates conduction block (Eidelberg et al. 1975). The exposure of fast voltage gated potassium channels clustered in the paranodal regions of myelinated axons by retrograde retraction of myelin away from the node also contributes to a

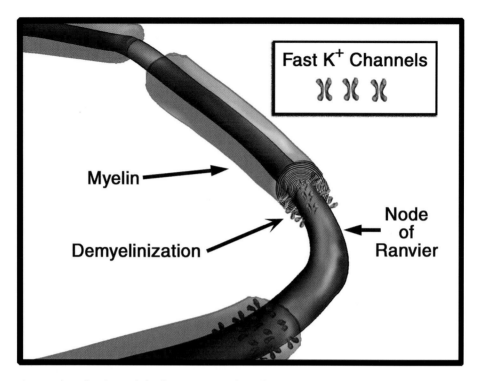

Fig. 13. Demyelination and the fast potassium channel. Fast potassium channels are clustered beneath the myelin sheath at paranodal regions of the nodes. Usually they are covered by the myelin at this region of specialized membrane (*foreground*). After injury, myelin may retract away from the nodes, exposing the channels in axons that survive the insult, or alternately produce poorly myelinated internodal regions. This creates a short circuit K^+ current when this region depolarizes, extinguishing the action potential before it can propagate across the nodal region. When 4-Aminopyridine blocks these voltage-gated, fast K^+ channels, it is believed this produces an increased action current and an increase in the duration of the action potential, leading to propagation of the depolarization wave across the internodal region. This figure suggests the likely mechanism of action whereby physiological recovery in poorly myelinated (or demyelinated) axons leads to functional recovery after SCI. The text outlines several other ways in which potassium channel blockade may enhance excitability and motorneuron functioning

local K^+ short circuit current squelching propagation of the nerve impulse across the node (Fig. 13). Reduction, even reversal, of this conduction block can be accomplished by K^+ channel blockade, in particular, using the fast potassium channel blocker 4 aminopyridine (4-AP). Over a decade ago, 4-AP was shown to facilitate electromyographical responses in paralyzed muscle during free fall in spinal rats (Blight and Gruner 1983; Blight 1989). Since the drug can be administered safely by intravenous injection or orally, use of potassium channel blockade as a clinical treatment for SCI was pioneered in our research center using naturally injured paraplegic dogs by veterinary surgeon, James Toombs, and physiologist, Andrew Blight (Blight et al. 1991). Variable levels and kinds of functions were recovered in chronically paraplegic dogs, sometimes within minutes after 4-AP injections. The recovery was independent of the months or years the animal had been paralyzed. Moreover, as the drug was metabolized, dogs returned to their original neurological status, thus serving as their own control. This veterinary clinical trial led to the first human clinical trials in collaboration with two Canadian medical centers, one led by Keith Hayes at The University of Western Ontario in London, Ontario and at McMaster University School of Medicine in Hamilton, Ontario, by neurosurgeon, Robert Hansebout (incidentally who nearly 2 decades earlier had conducted pioneering studies of hypothermia in spinal cord-injured patients) (Hayes et al. 1994; Hansebout et al. 1993). Presently, an oral form of the drug (fampridine) is in an advanced stage of human clinical testing in roughly 70 clinical centers in the US and Canada.

What is important to emphasize is that use of 4-AP is particularly important to long-term or chronic spinal injury. Since the amount and region within the spinal cord segment where white matter is left intact but nonfunctional is variable, the responses to 4-AP therapies in man and animal are likewise variable. Some people occasionally achieve remarkable improvement in motor and/or sensory functioning, respiratory control, incontinence, as well as reductions in spasticity, while others patients do not respond at all. For the persons in the middle, one might suppose that those who regain modest behavioral returns must decide if this represents sufficient improvements in the quality of their life to remain on the medication for what is likely to be the rest of their lives.

For some patients, there is a limit to the concentration of 4-AP sustainable in plasma, ultimately in cerebrospinal fluid (CSF) before unwanted side effects of the drug limit its usefulness. One can theoretically counter this by infusion of the drug directly into the CSF via the subarachnoid space of the spinal cord. We pioneered this technique in dogs using a telemetric indwelling pump to deliver 4-AP directly to CSF in collaboration with neurosurgeon, Kimbal Pratt, of Indiana University School of Medicine (Pratt et al. 1994). Though a promising variation of 4-AP therapy, there has not been a similar metered intrathecal delivery of the drug in human SCI. The only related test I am aware of was an inconclusive attempt at short-term (4–5 h) intrathecal infusion of the drug in only six patients using an externalized catheter (Halter et al. 2000). As it binds, or is somehow sequestered, in local regions of the subarachnoid space where it is introduced, 4-AP does not distribute throughout the CNS compartment (Pratt et al. 1994). Thus, it is required that the catheter be located very near or within the lesion. This was claimed in Halter et al. (2000), but it was also disclosed that if the catheter was not able to be advanced past the lumbar level, it was not. This short report does not reveal which of the six patients received the drug at the lesion and which did not. This was unfortunate since there were few untoward side effects from the short period of infusion, and in two patients, beneficial responses included modest recovery of volitional motor control and in one patient, some improvement in sensory function was reported.

Perhaps more importantly, this small pilot study revealed that the concentration of 4-AP in CSF can be responsible for reversing stable behavioral deficits. Since systemic potassium channel blockade (say in response to oral or IV administration) would excite the entire nervous system, there has been some question as to how much contribution to improved functioning is actually dependent on reversing conduction block at the level of the spinal injury. Intrathecal delivery is central to answering this question (Pratt et al. 1994). Recovery of even a few functions after intrathecal delivery in humans has in part answered in the affirmative. I have purposely oversimplified the probable mechanisms of systemic K⁺ channel blockade to intro-duce the reader to the concept. Of course there are other mechanisms that might work to promote functional recovery as well. For example, 4-AP may increase the ex-citability of internuncial neurons, particularly those that modify corticospinal path-ways, as well as a general facilitation of both CNS and PNS synaptic transmission (see Wolfe et al. 2001).

Most experimental therapies are aimed at interfering with the progression of the spinal injury in the acute phase. Novel approaches, such as offered by K⁺ channel blockade, for the long-term or chronically injured patient, are relatively few. So far, this technique is the only one, to my knowledge, being tested that has been clearly *proven* able to recover variable functions in people with long-standing injuries.

7.2
Repair

Interesting repair strategies for spinal cord injury are numerous. While the concept of restoration involves reviving physiological functioning in spared axons, repair strategies are aimed at reversing or stopping progressive destruction of the neural machinery at the lesion site. I prefer the term "repair" rather than "neuroprotection" for two reasons: (1) neuroprotection strategies are most often discussed in the con-text of cell body responses to damage and endogenous toxins. This is an important concept in brain injury, but not spinal cord injury, where the preservation of neurons may only marginally impact the recovery of clinical outcome measures, as discussed in Chap. 2, Sect. 2.2, "Characteristics of Spinal Cord Injury." In some of the repair strategies discussed below, the axolemmas that are damaged by secondary injury processes may spontaneously seal themselves if treated soon enough, while others may actually spontaneously restructure themselves to function normally. Thus, they are indeed "repaired" by the experimental treatment.

I have already discussed the concept of secondary injury. Historically this is the phase of SCI most vulnerable to attack by methods of repair. The use of methylpred-nisolone in human SCI was not based on its ability to reduce swelling, but mainly on animal data suggesting it was an effective free radical scavenger (Hall 1992). Another example of a hypothetical acute repair strategy involves interrupting the progressive destruction of the cytosol by unregulated ion exchange. We have discussed the cen-tral role of Ca^{++} entry into cells, truly a home-invasion homicide. Restricting unreg-ulated Ca^{++} entry by channel blockade seems to make sense, if it were clinically prac-ticable. However, the clinical use of Ca^{++} channel blockade in SCI has been both meager and inconclusive (Petitjean 1998) compared to extensive (and sometimes positive) testing for over 2 decades in cerebral stroke (Allen et al. 1983; Auer 1984; Gelmers 1984; Saveland et al. 1986). Numerous preclinical studies using animal mod-els of SCI have been conducted using numerous Ca^{++} blockers, including nimodip-ine, nicardipine, flunarizine, verapamil, diltiazem, and nifedipine. In two words I can summarize this SCI literature: very inconsistent.

The practical problem facing systemic Ca^{++} channel blockade secondary to SCI is that the desired reduction in secondary injury is compromised by numerous other actions, particularly in the vascular system. This is an especially important consider-ation in SCI, where blood pressure regulation and hypotension are critical management problems in many patients. On the face of it, the vasodilatory action of most Ca^{++} channel antagonists would be useful (Ross and Tator 1991), though this has been contested (Holtz et al. 1989). However, in practice, the compromised microcirculation of the spinal injury, the resultant problems in drug delivery to the lesion, and the level-dependent problem of reduced blood pressure (posttraumatic hypotension: the higher the vertebral injury level, the greater the problem), creates something of a morass for the SCI investigator. There is no clear modern data that suggest firmer ground has yet been reached.

Recall that Na^+ entry into cells also contributes to the release of intracellular Ca^{++} as well as depolarizing neuronal membranes. One might be able to both support more normal membrane potentials (thus excitability) and limit the progressive destruction of the neuron by Ca^{++}-mediated processes through the indirect means of interfering with Na^+ entry. Several intriguing reports over a 5-year period have explored the use of Na^+ channel blockade or poisoning as a means to improve functional outcome from SCI. One recent example (Rosenberg et al. 1999) provides very clear anatomical evidence for a reduction of white matter loss caused by SCI after treatment with tetrodotoxin. Moreover, this sparing was most evident in large caliber myelinated axons, those most susceptible to mechanical spinal cord injury (Blight and Decrescito 1986) and most characteristic of the failure to regenerate and form new connections.

There are numerous other physiological and biochemical anomalies occurring after CNS damage that play a role in secondary injury processes. These offer other avenues for clinical repair. Certain neurotransmitters such as glutamate and aspartate have been shown to increase in the extracellular microenvironment within minutes after SCI injury, and to be toxic to neurons at elevated concentrations under certain conditions. Various and specific membrane receptors such as N-methyl-D-aspartate (NMDA) and the DL-a amino-3-hydroxy-5-4 isoxazole, methylisoxazole propionic acid (AMPA) receptor have been implicated as important to the steady progression of SCI. Both of these receptors are specific to a class of agonist-mediated Ca^{++} channel gated by glutamate, and so are susceptible to glutamate endotoxicity. The net result, once again, is a mechanism of secondary injury implicated to increase intracellular Ca^{++} (see Wrathall et al. 1994). These putative mechanisms underlying the acute phase of injury then spin off experiments designed to interfere with them.

I do not believe, however, that the data support the view that reductionist understandings of cellular damage (NMDA, AMPA receptor antagonists, glutamate endotoxins, cytokine mediators, etc.) will lead to effective clinical treatments for SCI. It is becoming increasingly clear that many of these very potent biologically active molecules, including neurotrophic factors, produce a myriad of unwanted side effects in human patients. For example, intrathecal infusion of BDNF causes patients much difficulty, and NBQX, an AMPA/kainate receptor antagonist, is toxic to the liver. Furthermore, most of these approaches have bearing on cell death in neurons (neuroprotection strategies) and would only marginally impact the course of behavioral improvement in spinal cord-injured patients. As emphasized throughout this text, it is the disconnection in physiological conduction associated with broken white matter that is the crux of the problem in SCI.

Finally, there has arisen in the last 3 years another completely novel means of interrupting secondary injury processes. This involves the use of large hydrophilic polymers, surfactants, and nonionic detergents to immediately seal the initial breaches in cell membranes, rescuing the cell or its process from continuing dissolution. These techniques will be thoroughly detailed in sections to follow, as they are a focus of this monograph.

7.3
Regeneration

7.3.1
Peripheral Nerve Bridges

One of the earliest procedures used to produce CNS axonal regeneration was born of neurotransplantation techniques. Neurologists of the nineteenth century understood that, in part, it was the environment of the CNS that was implicated in the inability to sustain growth. Ramón y Cajal (1928) credits E. Lugaro with the first attempt to graft a sciatic nerve to the cerebrum to stimulate regeneration of central axons. This experiment failed, apparently because the grafts were too fresh, and time to sacrifice too short. Francisco Tello, however, tried again with older, degenerate, sciatic nerves and succeeded. *"These empty grafts, as Tello called them, are especially rich in neurotrophic substances."* (Ramón y Cajal 1928, p 739). The hollow segment of peripheral nerve trunks (that is, devoid of axons) were placed near previously made lesions of the cerebral cortex. Tello also placed grafts of Schwann cells undergoing division between the grafted peripheral trunk and the terminal ends of the proximal segments of severed pyramidal axons. These grafts helped sustain regeneration of the pyramidal tracts *"crossing the mesoderm scar and invading the transplanted nerves"* (Ramón y Cajal 1928, page 738). Regeneration of axons into these grafts was described, and as well, the participation of Schwann cells (that invaded the lesion from the peripheral environment) in this new growth of nerve fibers.

An inaccurate, and unfair, mythology has been recently created concerning the early use of peripheral nerve bridges in mammalian CNS experimentation. The myth explains that Wilfred Le Gros Clark's 1942 failure to repeat the results of Francisco Tello pushed the bridge experimentation into oblivion – forgotten and ignored until resurrected by Samuel David and Albert Aguayo in 1981 (read Schwab 1990, p 454; Schwab and Bartholdi 1996, p 335; and Vikhanski 2001, p 59). This sort of serially perpetuated inaccuracy robs the new student of an appreciation of the history of scientific investigation, and the orderly progression of methods and ideas driving critical experimentation. In fact, the use of peripheral nerve bridges had a very busy and very long history of experimentation after the days of Santiago Ramón y Cajal and Francisco Tello. Most of the time the results of PNS grafts into the CNS were positive. In one of the first detailed examinations of induced CNS regeneration after the turn of the nineteenth century (using several different methods), bridges fashioned from sciatic nerve were transplanted into the severed spinal cord of adult rats (Sugar and Gerard 1940). They wrote: *"The nerve implants served likewise as a growth bridge and new nerve fibers followed faithfully the path laid down by the degenerated ones (the sciatic graft), even when this curved back in a semicircle"* (p 9).

Sugar and Gerard in fact described the sciatic bridges as providing the best vehicle for regeneration of the three methods tested, including insertion of muscle fibers and implants of mashed brain or spinal cord. They state that *"peripheral nerve has long been used as a bridge to encourage neural regeneration"* (p 14), citing Tello and Ramón y Cajal but also Loez and Arcaute (1913) who bridged severed optic nerves. Investigation of PNS bridges inserted into brain or spinal cord of the mammal continued through the next 3 decades by Feigin et al. (1951); Yakovleva (1954); Campbell et al. (1960); Galabov (1966); Horvat (1966, 1980); Kao (1974); Heinicke (1978, 1980); and Chi et al. (1980) – an incomplete list at that.

Moreover, Le Gros Clark was not the only early investigator who could not replicate these findings: neither could Barnard and Carpenter (1950) nor Feigin et al. (1951). Most of these investigators, however, reported significant CNS nerve regeneration and a reduction in scarring when peripheral nerve tissue bridged CNS wounds. This latter observation lead Kao to report more robust regeneration if the bridge was inserted after a week's delay in dog spinal cord transections, and the scar tissue surgically removed prior to implantation (Kao et al. 1977). All of these studies evaluated axonal regeneration by the best techniques of the times, including electron microscopy in the 1970s. The true contribution of Samuel David, Albert Aguayo, and Peter Richardson, was the unambiguous formal proof that these early investigators were indeed correct. This was accomplished through the careful use of intracellular labels unavailable at the time to the others.

The Montreal group continued a long series of investigations using this venerable yet antique method to offer important modern insights into CNS regeneration (David and Aguayo 1985; Richardson et al. 1982; Richardson et al. 1984; Richardson and Issa 1984). One of the most splendid was the use of a segment of peripheral nerve to replace the optic nerve, reconnecting the eye with the superior colliculus of the hamster brain. Retinal ganglion cells projected regenerating axons through the graft to the brain, making synaptic contacts within the superficial layers of the superior colliculus. Not only were the bridges able to permit long-distance regenerative growth of CNS axons, but the synapses were electrophysiologically functional, mediating both inhibitory and excitatory postsynaptic responses to bursts of light presented to the eye (see Keirstead et al. 1989; Bray et al. 1987; Vidal-Sanz et al. 1987). As useful as these observations are to the student of the biology of CNS nerve regeneration in mammals, they have not proved to be useful in preclinical SCI experiments.

There was considerable excitement in the scientific and popular press over a report from Lars Olsen's group claiming to produce partial functional recovery after peripheral nerve bridge transplantations into a surgically produced gap in adult rat spinal cords (Cheng et al. 1996). Into this gap, 18 individual peripheral nerve bridges (derived from intercostal nerves) were claimed to have been inserted and glued in place with a fibrin adhesive containing fibroblast growth factor. Unbelievably, it was claimed that these grafts were connected such that descending pathways were redirected from the rostral white matter to gray matter of the caudal spinal cord segment, and ascending projections were routed from the caudal white matter to gray matter of the rostral segment. Documentation was not provided to establish that this daunting surgery was successful – especially when using such a large number of bridges placed within the small diameter of the rat cord. Clear anatomical evidence of CNS axons within any one bridge was not provided (only neurofilament staining which would mark CNS or PNS nerve processes). The claim of partial hind limb functional recovery in response to the transplantation technique was not convincing. The investigators used an open-field walking score as a behavioral test. The range was 0 (complete paralysis) to 5 (normal walking). Scores of 1 and 2 were defined by movement of the limbs that was not reflexive; however, it was not reported if this included forward locomotion or stepping. One might assume it did not, since a score of 3 noted active support and uncoordinated gait. Only four animals in the bridged groups were described as having achieved this grade. This proved to be significant compared to total paralysis (all scoring 0) for all controls for the entire period of observation.

First, movement in hind limbs in nonambulatory animals cannot be accepted as being based on anything but spinal reflexes unless data and details are provided to the contrary. Secondly, the total failure of any stepping whatsoever in control animals is not in accordance with the literature. Without more documentation, this report fails to meet a standard of proof for either regeneration or functional recovery. Characteristically, larger more informative reports usually appear subsequent to a preliminary telegraphic report in the journals *Science* or *Nature*. Unfortunately, the subsequent paper (Cheng et al. 1997) did not provide any further documentation of this controversial experiment, instead describing improvements in behavioral testing. To my knowledge, no one has ever duplicated this experiment.

7.3.2
Regeneration in Response to Neurotransplantation

Another technique with a long history, is the transplantation of fetal nervous tissue into the spinal cord lesion. Paul Reier and his colleagues, John Houle and Douglas Anderson, have produced a substantive literature on this topic (see Reier et al. 1988; Reier et al. 1992; Houle and Reier 1988, 1989; Giovanini et al. 1997; Friedman et al. 2000). Clear anatomical evidence supporting the long-term survival of these fetal grafts and the exchange of fibers (in growing host axons and efferent axons originating in the graft projecting into host parenchyma) have been provided. The integration of these grafts is much better in very young rats, and is less robust in fully adult ones, and both require immunosuppression to achieve transplant longevity. There are interesting differences between the type of embryonic tissue moved into the spinal cord and the type of axons that form synapses with it, though this detail is beyond the scope of this text. Thus, the notion that transplants of fetal nervous tissue might form patches or relays within the spinal cord lesion linking neuronal connections on either side is partly satisfied on anatomical grounds. The hypothesis that these protoplasmic kisses actually form electrophysiological relays is however, partially satisfied since electrical stimulation of dorsal roots adjacent to fetal grafts evoked postsynaptic potentials in the graft, revealing the capability of the grafts to form excitable, functional synapses with host neurons. The behavioral literature supporting the use of fetal transplants is problematic. Even if you grant the investigators the benefit of the doubt relative to behavioral testing and what it means (and I usually do not), a dilemma arises in that functional improvements in rats is reported to occur with all age groups so far transplanted with fetal tissues, from newborn to fully adult. Paradoxically, the best evidence for the maintenance of neural connections between graft and host occurs only in newborn or very young rodents. It seems unnecessary to dissect these functional studies further since fetal cell transplantation has already moved to human clinical testing in Florida. This is the most important endgame, the only test of real significance. So far, behavioral improvement still appears out of reach; however, the cysts that normally form in human SCI appear to become filled with the transplanted cells and their progeny. This information has been presented at meetings, but I do not know of a published preliminary report at this time. Altogether, the decades of hard work and exhaustive documentation of fetal cell transplantation by Paul Reier and his colleagues demands respectful attention. Of the clinically possible neurotransplantation techniques, this one has earned its place in human testing in spite of the public controversy concerning the acquisition and use of human embryonic tissues.

There are other numerous and varied types of transplant procedures in SCI animal studies. Examples include implants of Schwann cells (mainly to myelinate CNS axons, though this occurs normally), transplants of cells such as fibroblasts and Schwann cells (genetically engineered to produce nerve growth factor and other trophic substances; see Menei et al. 1998; Tuszynski et al. 1997; Nakahara et al. 1996; Grill et al. 1997), autogeneic transplants using a source of renewable neurons in the adult mammal (olfactory neurons and enteric neurons; Borgens et al. 1995), macrophage relocation/transplantation (see below in this section), hybridomas (as a continuous source of monoclonal antibodies such as IN-1), and the new celebrity cell type(s) stem cells. At this time, it is hard to prognosticate which of these might prove safe enough to move to human clinical trials in SCI though neoplastic cells are problematic, including genetically modified ones. I note a report that four patients will receive autogenic transplants of olfactory ensheating cells meant to improve remyelination of spinal white matter. The ethics of this plan has sparked controversy (see "Newsdesk", *The Lancet*, September 2002). This difference of opinion arises from the uneven results obtained in animals, and claims that Schwann Cell implants are more effective (Wewetzer et al. 2002; Takami et al. 2002; Ramon-Cueto and Santos-Benito 2001).

We in spinal cord injury sometimes develop tunnel vision, endlessly arguing about axonal regeneration or the lack of it, and if functional recovery in our animals is real or a masquerade. A postdoctoral fellow in our laboratory, himself a high-level quadriplegic, once cracked wise that a cure for him "would be to become a paraplegic". It takes you aback a bit to hear that. There are so many problems that require attention in SCI, sometimes improving voluntary locomotion is just not high on an injured person's list. One of the most challenging, sometimes unyielding issues is that of central pain – pain that can be lifelong and does not respond to drugs or other newer techniques such as afferent electrical stimulation. Interestingly, neurotransplantation techniques focusing on the treatment of pain seldom are considered in SCI reviews, but this is a fascinating subject and may help medicine turn the corner on this problem. For example, chromaffin cells of the adrenal medulla generate and secrete endogenous antipain substances: opioid peptides, metenkephalin, leuenkephalin, adrenergic transmitter substances, and other nociceptive modulatory neuropeptides. Transplantation of adrenal medulla tissues to animal models of central pain has shown real promise. Thus far these are xenographs that must be accompanied by immunosuppression, just as the fetal cells discussed in this section, usually with cyclosporin A. However, this science has moved even further and is now in small clinical trials using terminal patients with severe and intractable pain.

Adrenal tissues were obtained from organ banks, supported in culture for a week to confirm cell viability, and subsequently moved into the subarachnoid space, usually by lumbar puncture. Some of these patients remained pain-free after the transplantation. I recommend a different sort of review of these and other transplantation procedures by Jacqueline Sagen (1997), who recounts some of the same old subject matter, but with a different twist, and explores the efforts of her laboratory and others in the modification of pain through transplantation.

7.3.3
Stem Cells

All of the transplantation techniques mentioned (save pain) might meet the requirements for a treatment for SCI – but only likely through the relay hypothesis discussed in the preceding section. The production of new neurons per se in the gray matter lesion is likely to be of little significance (see Chap. 2, Sect. 2.2, "Characteristics of Spinal Cord Injury"). The potential use of neural stem cells is no different. Unless such cells form multitudinous neurites and synapses in host neural tissue, their hypothetical contribution to recovery is questionable.

Over a decade ago stem cells might have been called mesenchyme or germ cells, noting embryonic progenitor cells that, given the right instructions, can differentiate into cell lines of different phenotypes. The dream that developmental biology might actually harness the reparative, or regulative, power of the embryo is now perhaps becoming a reality. There is no question that replacing (through transplantation) nerve cells lost to disease and injury is of enormous importance, and may be side-stepping the issue of immunological rejection in the process. For a recent and informative review of the possibilities and problems facing this novel research, see Vescovi and Snyder (1999) and Smith (2001).

It is unquestioned that pluripotent neural stem cell lines can differentiate into the major types of CNS residents including neurons, astrocytes and oligodendrocytes, and that they can form stable populations in situ in the absence of neoplasms, as well as other uncontrollable outcomes (McDonald et al. 1999; Liu et al. 2000; Vescovi and Snyder 1999). In a new area of research such as this, many excellent researchers from other disciplines become enthusiastically involved, but are not seasoned in the peculiarities of SCI experimentation. In other cases, the reach of the report exceeds its experimental grasp. This is not helped by the drum beat of the popular media, whose attention to stem cells has recently become both loud and persistent. An example: the results of implantation of a D3-derived mouse stem cell line into compression injuries of the *rat* spinal cord. The behavioral scoring in this report was criticized earlier in Chap. 5, Sect. 5.1.1, "The BBB Evaluation," since recovery in injured spinal cord was claimed, even though the authors admitted that the improvement in stem cell-treated animals did not speak to the issue of improving conduction through the lesion (McDonald et al. 1999). Moreover, it is likely that it simply did not.

An example of the former (one of several reports from top-drawer tissue engineering laboratories) was already faulted in the same section for mishandling of the BBB behavioral scoring system (Vacanti et al. 2001). This report also provided a means of scoring sensory responses in stem cell-implanted mice (also on a 1–6 scale) that was summed with the modified BBB scale to provide a type of total neurological score. This sensory scoring system was just as problematic as the motor scoring method.

Animals were given a 0 for the complete lack of hind limb reflexes, considered a sensory test. Actually, this subgroup should have been eliminated from the study population if either transplanted or sham mice were indeed totally areflexic. Scores of 1 and 2 indicated reflex movements in one or both limbs, respectively. Such reflex movements should normally be present in all animals, even though 3 mm of their cord was removed beginning at T9. Scores of 3 and 4 indicated head turning toward an unspecified stimulation, while 5 and 6 indicated controlled limb withdrawal on one or both sides, respectively. These latter two grades could also be indicative of the withdrawal reflex that would be expected to be intact in all animals, independent of their treatment. What the term "controlled" meant, or how this test was conducted, was not described. With 4 of the 6 sensory grades devoted to, or complicated by, spinal reflexes that are normally functional after transection, validation of such a scoring procedure would normally be required as a separate report. These results also beg the question of why control animals faired so poorly in this testing, a common problem in SCI studies in rats and mice.

What is characteristic of all stem cell/SCI reports that I have studied is that they are heavy in experimental detail, particularly concerning identification of the various cells that may differentiate from the implanted cell line in situ. This component of these papers is worthwhile reading and informative. Unfortunately, I have not read even one report that clearly indicates a functional recovery from SCI secondary to implantation of stem cells.

Perhaps more importantly, what exactly do the proponents of stem cell implantation in the spinal cord expect to happen? Do they really wish to increase the numbers of astrocytes in the spinal lesion in addition to marked glial hyperplasia? As Silver points out, there are at least two classes of astrocytes that populate these lesions: one set produces significant problems for recovery of function (refer to Chap. 3, Sect. 3.1.1, "Other Inhibitors"). Do they really wish to increase the numbers of oligodendrocytes? One could argue this both ways; perhaps increased numbers of oligodendrocytes would enhance myelination. Perhaps increased oligodendrocytes would create an even more inhospitable microenvironment since there are claims that their membranes are replete with membrane proteins inhibitory of axonal regeneration. Even if we experimentally increase the numbers of neurons at the lesion site, their contribution to a recovery of function would be marginal.

There was a time when developmentalists such as myself learned about the potential for cellular differentiation in the adult mammal through studies of the ectopic, or better yet, de novo formation of skin, parts of the eye, and teeth developing inside ovarian cysts. Early on, many of us considered the prospect of stem cell implantation with real concern. Nowadays, molecular developmentalists are developing interesting techniques of phenotype control, narrowing the possibilities of uncontrolled or unregulated cell differentiation. My concern now, before a rush to human SCI pilot studies is: what is the expected outcome of adding these cells to the lesion, and what really is the rationale behind proposed recoveries of function secondary to spinal injury? There are plenty of stem cell lines available for testing in spinal cord injuries, but the logic behind their use seems in short supply.

My father, Col. Clarence Borgens, is in the final stages of a very grim, 25-year-long battle with Parkinson's disease. I am indeed optimistic that replacing specific neurons of the brain with neural stem cell-derived neurons may indeed reduce or eliminate his kind of suffering in generations to come. Not just for Parkinson's, but other injury and diseases of the brain where the death and loss of neurons is a central issue. I just do not see recovery from spinal cord injury in this same context.

7.3.4
Inhibiting the Inhibitors of Nerve Regeneration

Undoubtedly, the most cited research of the 1990s in the area of axonal regeneration in the mammalian CNS has been that of Martin Schwab and his colleagues at the Brain Research Institute in Zurich. I have already introduced the issue of endogenous blockers of axonal regeneration intrinsic to the mammalian CNS, particularly myelin-associated proteins found in the membranes of oligodendrocytes. It is clear that these proteins exist and interfere with nerve growth in vitro and this is an excellent series of studies by Schwab's group. Characteristic of the history of SCI experimentation, things begin to unravel when testing this interesting approach using in vivo and small animal models of SCI. This series of animal studies has become extraordinarily influential as part of the basic biology of CNS injury and, touted as a potential therapy in the clinic. Do these data hold up to such expectations on close inspection?

The earliest claims for axonal regeneration based on "inhibiting the inhibitors" was anatomically based. A monoclonal antibody to myelin associated inhibitory proteins (NI 250 and N 35) was developed (IN-1). IN-1 was delivered to rat spinal cord lesions by transplantation of the hybridomas that generated the antibodies in vitro. The hybridoma transplantation was performed at the same time as a partial transection of the spinal cord. It was claimed that the regeneration of descending corticospinal tracts in adult rat spinal cord was induced by blocking the action of these myelin inhibitory proteins (Schnell and Schwab 1990). I have already mentioned that the knowledge of where the ends of anterograde-labeled axons are in relation to the plane of transection of the cord is critical to evaluation of the success, or failure, of studies of axonal regeneration. In the first report of this series, a marker device was reported to have been inserted into the cord to determine the plane of transection. However, the report did not provide documentation of the use of the device, the plane of transection established by it, the relative location of the terminals of control and treated axons relative to this identified plane, or even the existence of clear terminals themselves (Schnell and Schwab 1990). After the short report in the journal *Nature*, use of the marker was apparently abandoned in a subsequent full paper (Schnell and Schwab 1993) and another short report comparing corticospinal tract "regeneration" facilitated by three neural growth factors: brain-derived neurotrophic factor (BDNF), nerve growth factor (NGF), and neurotrophins-3 (NT-3) to IN-1 (Schnell et al. 1994).

I will go further and opine that the documentation in this series of reports does not support the claim of axonal regeneration of the corticospinal tract. Instead, these data reveal a possible effect on collateral sprouting. The extension of corticospinal fibers around the lesion in the ventral cord could just as easily have been due to collateral sprouting from intact fibers below the plane of the dorsal hemisection. Collateral sprouting, as discussed, is not axonal regeneration. Schwab and colleagues did not trace the route of individual labeled axon(s) arising from the severed corticospinal tract into the caudal spinal cord segment in any of these reports. Moreover, the claim of axonal regeneration was undercut by the description of *"massive sprouting at the lesion site in the controls"* (Schnell and Schwab 1990 p 272) and *"spontaneous sprouting of the lesioned CST fibers occurred at all three levels"* at the lesion, and 1 and 4 mm from it (Schnell et al. 1994, p 171). The use of very young rats in all of these experiments does not bode well for the contention that axonal regeneration was induced by IN-1 treatment, but rather sprouting (2- to 6-week-old rats, Schnell and Schwab 1990; 3- to 4-week-old rats, Schnell and Schwab 1993; 4- to 7-week-old rats in Schnell et al. 1994). The regenerative growth of axons can still be robust in 2- to 3-week-old rats. As Martin Berry reviews, a typical mature CNS scar does not even begin to form in response to injury in the rat cord until about the second postnatal week, and this is likely associated with the endogenous powers of axonal regeneration seen in younger rodents (Berry 1979). Schwab and colleagues did not segregate their data, separating the youngest of the rats studied (2–3 weeks postnatal) from the older ones. In my opinion, this likely would have revealed an age-dependent character in the axonal responses to IN-1, favoring an enhancement of collateral sprouting and not axonal regeneration.

Throughout this series of papers, all employing partial transection of the spinal cord, the extensions of corticospinal axons into the caudal segment was variously described as regeneration, sprouting, regenerative sprouts, or simply "sprouts". Perhaps because the issue of sprouting versus regeneration could not be resolved, subsequent studies investigated CNS plasticity (the normal ability of the CNS to remodel itself after damage) where such distinctions did not have to be made. Two recent anatomical studies have suggested that the limited sprouting that occurs in response to brain lesions in fully adult rats was increased by IN-1 applications (1- to 2-month-old rats in Kartje et al. 1999 and Wenk et al. 1999). Unfortunately, enthusiasm for these anatomical data is dampened by the very indirect means of documentation by a densitometry-based method instead of careful morphometry. An earlier report claimed functional recovery from pyramidal lesions in adult rats as well. Though the behavioral tests used in this study were inventive, the results and interpretation contained in this report were fundamentally flawed.

For 3 weeks before pyramidotomy, rats were trained to perform a series of tasks such as reaching for food pellets, walking on grids, and rope climbing. The mean scores for these various outcome measures were not compared between the experimental and control groups. The foundation of the claim of behavioral recovery was instead based upon comparisons of posttreatment behavioral scores with the prelesioning scores achieved by the same animals within each group. In the absence of a direct comparison of the outcome data between groups, these results are not convincing. When one looks more closely at the raw data when provided, the unease with the author's conclusions grows. For example, rats were trained to grasp and eat food pellets, a task which was scored before injury in both controls and IN-1-treated rats. The authors state that this capability was significantly decreased from a success rate of 19 of 20 pellets grasped and eaten for both control *and* experimental animals before spinal injury to a success rate of approximately 16 of 20 in the control groups (lesion only and anti-HRP controls) by 42 days after the operation (Z'Graggen et al. 1998). Recovery to pretreatment success levels were claimed for the IN-1-treated animals. It is likely, however, that the injury did not produce a change in the success rate for animals performing this task. There is not a proportional difference between 19 successes in 20 attempts compared to 16 successes of 20 attempts ($P=0.34$; Fisher's exact test, two-tailed), and it is difficult to see how statistical significance could be reached had the mean success rates been compared between the groups (which they were not).

Other laboratories have tried to corroborate these results. *Unfortunately*, spotty labeling of antereogradely filled fibers distal to an *incomplete* transection of the cord (Bergman et al. 1995) is unconvincing support for the claims of "long distance" regrowth of corticospinal axons. Reflex responses in the young rat hindlimbs are likewise insufficient data to support claims of an SCI "recovery" in the absence of a clear validation of supraspinal control.

In summary, there is little to no unambiguous evidence to support the claim of induced axonal regeneration in spinal cord in response to inhibiting myelin-associated protein with a monoclonal antibody raised against it. The behavioral data suggesting a recovery of function from SCI based on a similar premise is so far very uneven.

7.3.5
Do Macrophages Hurt or Help Regeneration in the Spinal Cord?

At the outset, the notion that macrophages can induce axonal regeneration seems something of a rhetorical oxymoron. If anything, their phagocytic occupation, their voracious, aggressive migration into wound to debride them, and their secretion of numerous hydrolytic, and other catabolic enzymes would seem to spell disaster for whatever healthy cells remained in the environment that they invade. This may not be entirely true, however. In a unique twist, several investigators have put forward the notion that setting the conditions to be favorable for nerve regeneration requires a robust inflammatory reaction, and that some of the cytokines liberated by activated macrophages can act as growth factors. Macrophages are indeed little cytokine factories and secrete numerous proinflammatory cytokines into the microenvironment. Some of these, such as interleukin-6 (IL-6), appear to benefit the CNS injury (Klusman and Schwab 1997), perhaps by antagonizing the deleterious effects of cytokines IL-1 and tumor necrosis factor (Schindler et al. 1990). There are indeed interesting experiments such as Prewitt et al. 1997 that provide some direct evidence for the notion of macrophage-facilitated regeneration in spinal cord. Furthering the view of the beneficial role of macrophages in the inflammatory stage of neural repair holds that macrophage infiltration into CNS wounds is late in arriving and anemic compared to an early, robust inflammatory reaction in peripheral nerve injuries. This suggested to some investigators that the failure of CNS regeneration might be related to this difference (George and Gariffin 1994; Perry and Brown 1992; Perry and Gordon 1988; Perry et al. 1993). Transplantation of macrophages, activated in peripheral nerve injuries, into transected optic nerve lesions was associated with increased axonal regeneration (Lazarov-Speigler 1996).

On the other hand, there is evidence that macrophages may be responsible for substantial death and secondary injury, particularly in spinal cord and brain injury, based on the introductory statements in the preceding paragraph, and so-called bystander damage. "Bystander damage" (Andrew Blight's description) is collateral damage associated with simply the numbers of accumulating macrophages during the inflammatory stage of CNS wounds (Blight 1985, 1992; Giulian et al. 1989). In support of this notion is that reducing macrophages through various means such as the administration of a macrophage toxin (silica) improves behavioral outcome from CNS injury (Blight 1994; see also Giulian and Robertson 1990). The members of each of these camps do not seem to want to go after each other in print, one group attempting to accommodate the views of the other by shifting the focus from the central injury to more distant regions of Wallerian degeneration of white matter, and then returning. Unfortunately, for such good will and collegiality, macrophages are either supportive of axonal regeneration in the CNS or they are not. Secondly, the suggestion that macrophages are few in number and late in arriving in CNS wounds compared to PNS wounds is a testable one.

Our laboratory has always been impressed with the sheer numbers of these cells migrating into the spinal cord lesion during the first 10 days or so after injury, reaching densities of nearly 6,000 cells/mm^2 (Moriarty and Borgens 1999). This density reminds me of a benign tumor whose very presence squeezes out normal cells, totally supporting the concept of bystander damage. Furthermore, there is little quantitative support for the notion of a late or anemic immigration of macrophages into CNS wounds (reviewed by Leskovar et al. 2000). A recent evaluation of monoclonal-labeled activated macrophages using computer-based morphometry (where there was no human interaction in the generation of numerical data) has provided an answer to this question. Macrophage densities were determined in crushed spinal cord and crushed sciatic nerve in the same animal at the same time points after injury. These cell counts did not support the notion of a late and sparse macrophage accumulation in spinal cord. Macrophages not only moved into spinal wounds earlier and in statistically significantly greater densities than in the PNS wounds, but their production of proinflammatory cytokines was up-regulated earlier than was measured in the injured sciatic nerve (Leskovar et al. 2000).

Finally, I do not believe that optic nerve lesions (often used as a model for CNS regeneration), as performed in Lazarov-Speigler 1996, are particularly relevant to spinal cord injuries, even though these CNS axons may share a reduced capacity to regenerate. Lesions to the cord result in a massive hemorrhagic contusion injury and dramatic secondary injury phenomenon. A crush injury to the optic nerve does not produce such wholesale destruction of tissue associated with a massive and spreading lesion. Moreover, the inflammatory reaction in supraspinal CNS wounds is generally weaker than in spinal cord (Schnell et al. 1999).

Nonetheless, under the leadership of Michelle Schwartz, an experimental macrophage "therapy" has already moved into human testing. It is questionable if the clinical trials involving autogeneic transplantation of peripherally activated macrophages into human spinal cord injuries (conducted at Israel's Weizman Institute) is anything but premature. This rush to human implementation was conducted even though the literature on the biological role of macrophages in CNS and PNS regeneration is inconclusive and the supportive animal experimentation for such a clinical trial is scant. It is just possible that adding more phagocytes to the injury could worsen the outcome rather than help it – and this could also be something of a time bomb. Backing away only somewhat from my more enthusiastic love of a good war in the literature (which always seems to advance our understanding faster and further), there are indeed many mysteries concerning the role of macrophages in CNS injury. A spinal cord injury is not a static one after the acute period has passed. A spinal cord injury is a dynamic one throughout the life of an individual who sustains it. Macrophages can still be found in people's spinal injuries many years after their accident. A chronic spinal cord injury may be more like a chronic infection than a stable and healed wound in the skin. We have identified giant multinucleated macrophages inhabiting the spinal cord injury in rats, but not in peripheral nerve injuries. Such curious giant cells are indicative of chronic CNS disease and infection (like Alzheimer's disease or parasitic infections of the brain) and their appearance in the spinal lesion is both unexpected and unexplained (Leskovar et al. 2001).

7.3.6
The Neural Growth Factors

Various and many growth factors have been administered to spinal and brain injuries in numerous ways from continuous metered delivery by indwelling pumps (inosine by osmotic pumps; Benowitz et al. 1999) to the implantation of genetically engineered cells (such as fibroblasts engineered to produce NGF, BDNF, and other neurotrophic factors; Tuszynski et al. 1997; Nakahara et al. 1996; Blesch et al. 2002). This is a large and growing literature and beyond the scope of this review. One can conclude that there is indeed evidence for clear facilitation of axonal regeneration in response to the neurotrophins. I have been most impressed with the photomicrographs of nearly hair-like neurite extensions from brain neurons induced by Neurotrophic factors secreted by genetically engineered fibroblasts grafted into adult rat brain. Most growth factors are a subclass of cytokines, extraordinarily potent molecules producing varied responses in animals and man. We need to adopt a realistic view of delivery vehicles and method of gene regulation in this "new" discipline. In animals this has been accomplished by implantation of tumor cell lines (hybridomas) or genetically engineered cells that secrete neurotrophic factors such as BDNF or NGF. Some of the latter techniques have been applied to humans with terminal conditions and exhausted avenues of therapy such as amyotrophic lateral sclerosis. Possible unwanted side effects and unexpected outcomes (such as stimulation of latent neoplasms) has been a cloud hanging over human clinical application of the molecular based therapies. It is not likely that some of these techniques will be used in seriously injured people, who otherwise would enjoy a normal life expectancy after rehabilitation, until these issues are better understood and openly discussed. Furthermore, the many proponents of "gene therapy" for SCI should critically evaluate these potential problems rather than fail to even raise the issue (Lindsay et al. 1994; Blesch et al. 2002).

8 Biologically Produced Electrical Fields: Physiology Spoken Here

Like many other areas of developmental biology, an appreciation of the molecular and genetic controls of nerve growth and regeneration has dominated the last 40 years of inquiry. These approaches have indeed provided some stunning new insights, but they have also squeezed out other important disciplines. This intellectual myopia is particularly true concerning the literature on endogenous and applied voltages in development and regeneration. Other scholars have remarked upon this bias. Dale Purves and Jeff Lichtman noted in their book *Principles of Neural Development*: *"The idea that embryonic currents influence axon outgrowth (or other aspects of embryonic pattern) is often given rather short shrift"* (p 127).

I have often heard the complaint that "no one knows how electrical fields work," the unspoken pretense being that there is a broader and deeper understanding of how neurotrophins or neurotransplants work. This is nonsense. Actually, there is as much of a fundamental understanding of direct current (DC) electrical field effects on cells as any of the biochemistries of developmental control.

I think part of the problem has been that the term "electrical field" or "bioelectricity" seems to put many biologists off. Bioelectricity is not Kirlian photography, extrasensory perception, or something akin to carrying a magnet in your pocket to keep arthritis from flaring up. *Rather, one should reflect upon the deeper truth that all life processes are based upon electrical factors.* Whether it is the potential difference or voltage gradient (other synonyms for an electrical field) that is expressed across a cell membrane, the transepithelial potential (TEP) expressed across all epithelia, the dynamic phenomenon of nerve impulse conduction, or the transduction of environmental stimuli by receptors, all we are really talking about in cells, tissues, and animals is the science of physiology.

The study of physiology is dominated by electrical factors where current is carried by ions, and voltage gradients are always associated with the movement or separation of electrical charge:

1. The flow of electric current through cells and tissues is established by the movement of ions (and not electrons) in body fluids.
2. The fluids and tissues through which the current flows possess a measurable electrical resistance (resistivity; the mathematical inverse of conductance).
3. The gradient of voltage over the distance the current is flowing (through this resistance) is the electrical field or voltage gradient given by nothing more complicated than Ohms law ($V=iR$).

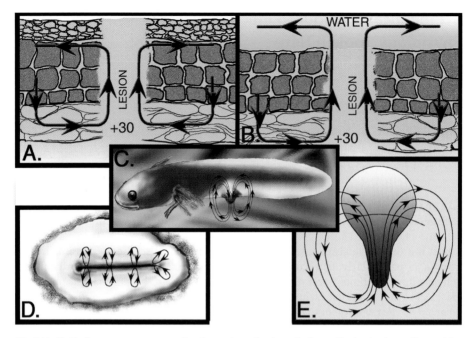

Fig. 14A–E. Endogenous currents and voltages in animals and plants. In **A**, the inwardly positive (approximately +30 mV) skin battery drives ionic current out of a skin wound. The return leg of the circuit is through the extracellular fluids of the apical living layers of skin, beneath the cornified layer. This can result in large lateral voltage gradients on either side of the wound (refer to Barker et al. 1982; Vanable 1989). In **B**, another wound is shown in amphibian skin. Similarly, current is driven out of the wound by the inwardly positive skin battery. The return leg of the circuit is through the pond water or moisture on the surface of the skin in semi-terrestrial or aquatic amphibians (see Borgens et al. 1977). In both cases, the current and voltage gradients produced by wounding are involved in skin wound healing, or in some species, regeneration of the extremity (reviewed by Borgens 1989). In **D**, currents are driven through the lateral walls of the primitive streak in the chick embryo (refer to Jaffe 1981), and in **C**, ionic currents predict the region of the formation of limbs in amphibian larvae (Borgens et al. 1983) and in mouse and chick embryos. In the latter, interruption of these currents by reversing their polarity with microelectrodes for approximately 5 h induced limb malformation seen about 1 week later (Altizer et al. 2001). In **E**, current enters the presumptive rhizoid of the fucus egg prior to the two-cell stage. Fucus is a diecious brown algae, whose initial polarity is set by light acting on the membrane to produce a transcellular ionic current. This initial polarity, leading to the thallus and rhizoid at the two-cell stage, can be overridden by several means,

8.1
Concerning Naturally Produced DC Voltage Gradients

Risking oversimplification for useful instruction, the mechanisms of the biological action of DC fields on cells falls into three overlapping categories: (1) extracellular voltages (endogenous or artificially applied) that exert their influence across the outside domain of cells (the extracellular face of membranes), and (2) across the cell membrane. A response to the former might be the lateral electrophoresis of charged components (such as receptors) floating in the plasmalemma leading to receptor capping. The latter can lead to hyperpolarization or depolarization of the cell membrane, depending on the polarity of the applied voltage. Finally, (3) the type of ion(s) carrying the current can grossly affect cell function and anatomy.

The convention established by Benjamin Franklin is that we define the direction of current flow as being in the direction in which positive charge will move. Thus, since a cell membrane is internally negative (by 50–90 mV) relative to the outside, a hole in the membrane (or a local area of low resistance in the membrane) will lead to net current entering the hole. Since most all animal skins are internally positive (by about 30–60 mV; Borgens 1982) relative to the outside, net electric (ionic) current will leave the wound (Fig. 14). Consider the possibly catastrophic effects on the cell if a steady Ca^{++} current enters it, leading to the accumulation of this ion in cytoplasm. Also appreciate that the voltage that naturally exists across either the cell membrane or the skin, in these examples, is indeed comparable to a battery. This battery will drive electric (ionic) current through the circuit established by the wound (Borgens 1977; Borgens 1989) until it runs down (depolarized and collapsed) or the hole in the cell membrane or skin is anatomically (i.e., electrically) sealed (Shi and Pryor 2000; Shi et al. 2000; Krause et al. 1994). Thus, it is both instructive and convenient to consider that natural DC bioelectricity can have both (1) voltage-mediated effects (in points 1 and 2 above in this section) and (2) current-mediated effects (as in 3 above), though they are inextricably linked in many cases.

To steal the old joke that location is the *three* most important considerations governing real estate – when it comes to endogenous or applied voltages, it is geometry, geometry, geometry. I say this even before we consider the magnitude of the natural or artificially imposed voltage. If the extended cell process (an axon) is 1 cm in length and is aligned parallel with the long axis of an imposed extracellular electrical field (1 V/cm), then the full potential drop of 1 V will be expressed across the 1-cm-long expanse of cell membrane. If, on the other hand, the axon is aligned perpendicular to the field, than the relatively minute cross-sectional area of that axon (ca. a few micrometers square) will be exposed to the fall in electrical potential. Thus, long cell processes oriented parallel with the gradient of voltage would be more likely to be penetrated or influenced by the voltage drop than if they are aligned perpendicular. The mathematical relationship governing the relative resistance of the membrane and cytoplasm to the flow of ionic current through or around the cell can be found in consideration of cable theory in neurophysiology. It is beyond the scope of this text to recite these principles; however, it is indeed the geometry of the cell exposed to the electrical field that is crucial to the probability that the cell can physiologically or anatomically respond.

Secondly, the arrangement of cells in relation to each other is an additional critical geometry to consider. The larger the extracellular space between cells (i.e., the larger the cross-sectional area of this region through which extracellular current must flow), the lower the resistance to the flow of current, and by Ohms law, the lower the associated voltage gradient in the extracellular space. The more densely packed the cells are (i.e., the less cross-sectional area of extracellular space through which the same magnitude of current must flow), the larger the current density, hence the electrical field. The relationship between the voltage gradient (in V/cm), the resistivity of the body fluids, cytoplasm, etc. (given in Ω cm), and the current density (in amps/cm^2) is indeed Ohms law for extended media (V/cm=A/cm^2 × Ω cm). Thus, considerations of geometry are critical to how one even begins to consider the biological effects of applied voltages, or endogenous transcellular or transtissue voltages and currents. Such considerations are conventional themes to the physiologist; for example, the measurements of extracellular voltage and current flow between retinal photo receptors using microelectrodes as in the classic measurements of the dark current (Hagins 1972).

To depolarize a nerve axon sufficient for it to fire an action potential using surface electrodes requires a considerable voltage to be applied to the cell, sometimes on the order of volts per millimeter. Most of the developmentally important voltages we will be discussing are orders of magnitude below that required to activate excitable cells. We will be considering electrical fields on the order of microvolts per millimeter to hundredths of millivolts per millimeter. Endogenous voltage gradients typically range from tenths of millivolts per millimeter to 1 V/mm, such as the transneural tube potential (TNTP) expressed across the developing neural tube (Shi and Borgens 1994).

Voltage gradients on this order can indeed change the anatomy and physiology of cells in predictable ways. First, we will consider the arrangement of membrane receptors, even ion channels, suspended in the membrane, and/or spanning it. These moieties have a net charge exposed to the extracellular domain and thus can be responsive to extracellular gradients of voltage. Certainly, weak applied fields can polarize the distribution of receptors on the cell surface. The first unambiguous demonstration of such lateral electrophoresis was the movement of decorated concanavalin A receptors redistributed within muscle cell membrane exposed to electrical fields (Poo and Robinson 1977).

An increasing restriction of ion channels such as Ca^{++} to a localized region on the growth cone provides a neat mechanism for possibly redirecting nerve fiber growth. Receptors for neurotrophins may cluster on the cathodal face of the growth cone, which is consistent with observations of greater filopodia activity on this face as well. Ca^{++} channels may distribute to the cathodal facing membranes of the growth cone facilitating Ca^{++} entry, filopodia activity, substrate adhesion (Gunderson and Barrett 1980), and finally turning of the neurite towards the cathode (McCaig 1989).

8.2
The Skin Battery and Electric Embryos

Before describing the regenerative responses of nerve fibers to artificially applied electric fields in adult mammals or the mechanisms of action underlying these responses, one should first consider why nerves might respond to such electrical cues in the first place. The answer likely resides in the fact that endogenous voltages play a role in morphogenesis in early neural development.

Physiologically produced voltage gradients are critical to a variety of developmental events in vertebrates. It is beyond the scope of this section to review all of these; however, the following list may direct the interested reader to this literature that includes wound healing (Vanable 1989), amphibian regeneration (Borgens 1989; Jenkins et al. 1996), the development of limbs in early vertebrate embryos (Borgens 1984; Altizer et al. 2001; Fig. 14), and the development and repair of nervous system components, the subject of the next two sections.

First, the ectoderm (and later the integument of the adult) of all vertebrates possesses a potential difference across itself, which is usually inwardly positive by some

30–90 mV. This potential difference occurs in association with the insertion of non-voltage gated ion channels in the apical layers of this developing syncytium. The ectoderm of embryos and the integument of adult animals can be thought of as being nearly identical in this regard. These channels allow the separation of ions between the interstitial environment within the embryo and their outside aqueous world, or in terrestrial animals, the moist apical surface beneath the cornified layers of the skin. Mostly, it is a nonvoltage gated Na^+ channel facilitating the inwardly directed diffusion of Na^+ from the outside milieu through the cells of the apical layers of the integument to be pumped into deeper interstitial regions by the ATP-dependent ion pumps of the basal membranes. This produces a transepithelial potential (TEP). The specific channels in ectoderm and skin responsible for the TEP have been characterized and are sensitive to a family of blocking agents typified by the diuretic amiloride (and similar compounds such as benzamil and the methyl-ester of lysine) (Kirschner 1973). This nonvoltage gated Na^+ channel is often referred to in the literature as the "amiloride sensitive sodium channel". Channel blockers such as amiloride and benzamil reversibly collapse the TEP when applied to the apical surface of ectoderm or skin. Apparently larval amphibian skin and embryonic ectoderm can eventually adapt to a chronic blockade, by pumping other ions. This adaptive movement of ions once again supports a TEP of the correct polarity (see Borgens et al. 1983). In all embryonic integuments that I am aware of (broadly defining the embryo's ectoderm as an integument as well), such a TEP is established very early, well before gastrulation. Ann Warner (1985) has suggested that the inward movement of Na^+ in the blastula carries with it water, which osmotically swells the blastocoele, inflating it into a round ball. It is also clear that in both anuran and urodele embryos, the magnitude of the ectodermal TEP increases with time after gastrulation (Robinson and Stump 1982; Shi and Borgens 1995).

Given that a substantial TEP resides across embryonic epithelium, any low-resistance region can then produce a leakage of ionic current through this pathway (recall the convention that the direction of current flow is defined as the direction in which positive charge will move). The smaller and more localized the current leak pathway, the more intense the current density passing through it from inside the embryo, and hence, the electrical field in this direction (Fig. 14).

Permit one example, the aforementioned limb bud current which predicts the exact position of limb emergence many developmental stages prior to even mesenchyme accumulation in frog (Robinson 1983), salamander (Borgens et al. 1983), and chick and mouse embryos (Altizer et al. 2001). The anatomy of this leak pathway has best been explored in the relatively slowly developing neoteneous axolotl larvae (Borgens et al. 1983). There is a localized breakdown of tight junctions in the flank ectoderm where limbs will form, days prior to limb bud formation. This induces outward current flow through this region, iniating a positive feedback loop causing even further dissolution of the organized anatomy of the flank integument in the region where the limb bud will emerge, revealed by ultrastructural investigation (Borgens et al. 1987). One report suggested limb bud currents in the amphibian were due to inward current at the gill, producing a complete circuit, balancing outwardly directed current at the limb forming region (Robinson 1983). This conclusion is in error since ionic currents at the gill (involved with osmoregulation in larval amphibians) are pumped across the gill in both directions. Such net current is variable in polarity, depending as it does on the balance of cations and anions transported at any given time. Moreover, there is no gill in the chick or mouse embryo at the stage of hind limb development, yet all of these vertebrate embryos drive prophetic currents out of limb-forming regions that are amiloride sensitive (Altizer et al. 2001). Indeed, the currents driven through embryos are generated by skin batteries.

8.2.1
Endogenous Voltages During Neurulation

More relevant to the emerging nervous system is a natural leakage pathway at the blastopore where ionic current driven by the ectodermal TEP leaves the embryo, completing the circuit through its watery domain (Fig 15A). Such currents can be measured without touching the embryo (or for that matter, a cell) with an extracellular vibrating electrode (Jaffe and Nucitelli 1974). The substantial densities of current pass through the embryo in a rostral-caudal direction and help polarize the early embryo fore to aft. The subectodermal head region of vertebrates is thus positive with respect to the tail region (where current exits at the blastopore). The fall in potential can be as high as 80–100 mV over 1 mm in the approximately 2-mm-long axolotl embryo (Fig. 14). Over the entire embryo, voltage gradients are on the order of 20 mV/mm, as sampled by microelectrode (Metcalf et al. 1994; Shi and Borgens 1995) (Fig. 15B).

This fall in voltage not only electrically polarizes the embryo, but anatomically polarizes it as well. Using the blastopore as a tail marker, we have aligned gastrulating urodele embryos in special chambers nose-to-tail, and imposed a voltage gradient across as many as 20 embryos at a time. By artificially manipulating the slope of the subectodermal voltage gradient (also monitored with microelectrodes), one can predictably alter either the morphology of the emerging head or tail depending on the slope of the voltage gradient imposed within the embryos by this procedure (Metcalf and Borgens 1994; Fig. 16).

Using both one- and two-dimensional extracellular noninvasive electrodes (the latter measures the vector of current entering or leaving a source), our laboratory discovered a second leak pathway at the margins of the rostral neural folds, measured in both anuran and urodele embryos (Borgens 1989; Metcalf et al. 1994). This leakage of current produces a fall in electrical potential within the neural plate of the embryo from the midline to the left and to the right. These gradients were measured using conventional microelectrode techniques (Fig. 15B). The vector of these gradients of voltage would be in the dorsal/ventral axis, leading to the possibility that one of the earliest three-dimensional blueprints for the body plan of early vertebrates is electrical, predating – perhaps helping to establish – the molecular/genetic blueprint (Shi and Borgens 1995). Furthermore, this three-dimensional coordinate system is expressed at the beginning of neurulation (at axolotl stage 14) and disappears at the beginning of neural tube formation (stage 20). Only during these critical stages can manipulation of the voltages by externally applied electrical fields induce predictable changes in the developmental anatomy of embryos (Jenkins and Borgens, unpublished observations; see also Metcalf and Borgens 1994).

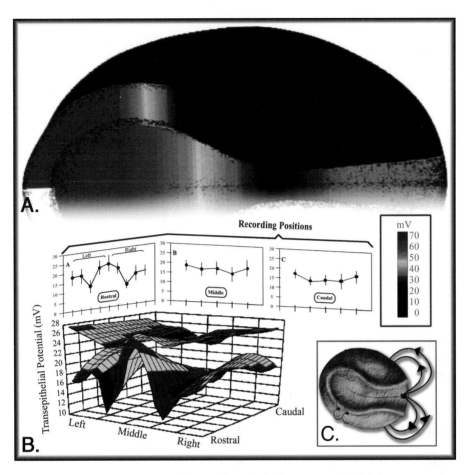

Fig. 15A–C. Endogenous voltages and the vertebrate body plan. A transepithelial (i.e., transectodermal) voltage of about 20–50 mV exists across the ectoderm of vertebrate embryos. This embryonic TEP has been measured in amphibians, avians, and mammals (and, incidentally, the embryos of numerous invertebrates). In the vertebrate embryo, the distribution of the TEP is not homogeneous. One can sample the magnitude of the TEP with a microelectrode referenced to the external milieu. If two samples, 1 mm apart, are both 20 mV in size, then there is no subectodermal voltage gradient between them. On the other hand, if a TEP of 20 mV is sampled at one location, and 50 mV 1 mm from it, then a subectodermal potential difference of 30 mV exists between them, producing a subectodermal electrical field (voltage gradient) of 30 mV/mm. A montage of such transepithelial measurements made in axolotl embryos is presented in this figure. At the top (**A**), a *pseudocolor scale* shows a substantial electrical field exists along the head/tail axis in the early neurula (head to the *left*, tail to the *right*). Vertebrate embryos at this early stage of neural development are positive at the head and negative at the tail, with potential drops in this direction as high as 70 mV/mm, and averaging 20–30 mV/mm over the entire animal along this axis. This voltage gradient is produced by a transembryo flow of ionic current, leaving the blastopore (*inset* **C**). At the margins of the neural folds on both sides of the midline – and more prominent in the rostral half of the embryo – a steady endogenous current is driven out of the lateral walls of the neural folds (*inset* **C**) through another low-resistance pathway. This produces a fall in electrical potential from the midline to the right, and

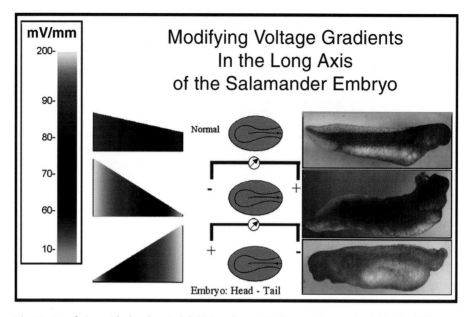

mV/mm

200-

90-

80-

70-

60-

10-

**Modifying Voltage Gradients
In the Long Axis
of the Salamander Embryo**

Normal

- +

+ -

Embryo: Head - Tail

Fig. 16. Interfering with the electrical field interferes with the morphogenetic field. The fall in potential from the positive head region of the embryo to the negative tail was shown in Fig. 15. Numerous axolotl embryos were aligned in specially constructed chambers head-to-tail and immersed in pond water. An artificially applied voltage gradient could be imposed across all of them using a DC power source and electrodes. The induced change in the slope of the endogenous subectodermal voltage gradient was sampled using microelectrodes. The *top row* shows the normal head/tail slope of this endogenous voltage gradient in a control animal developing in the chamber, but not in the presence of an imposed DC electrical field (compare to Fig. 15A). The orientation of the embryo, neural plate to the *left*, is shown in the icon. The photograph to the immediate *right* is typical of such a normally developing axolotl larvae. The *second row* shows the resultant voltage gradient produced when an electrical field is imposed across all embryos in the chamber: the negative pole at the head, positive pole at the tail. The *pseudocolor graph* reveals that in such cases, the slope of the natural voltage gradient is strikingly enhanced, hyperpolarizing the head end, depolarizing the tail ectoderm, but not affecting its polarity. Such a modification of the embryo's internal endogenous voltage gradient produced gross abnormalities to the developing head and brain, while the tail region of the embryo was largely unaffected. In the *bottom row*, the opposite polarity of the imposed electrical field produced the opposite response. The head region was depolarized, while the tail ectoderm was hyperpolarized; thus the polarity of the head/tail voltage gradient was reversed from normal. Such embryos developed head structures that were normal, while tails were structurally incomplete and misshapen. These responses to imposed fields were predictable, revealing head/tail morphogenesis to be dependent on a polarized internal electrical field

————————————————————————————————▶

Fig. 17A–D. The transneural tube potential and cranial development. The genesis of the transneural tube potential (*TNTP*) is shown in A and B. In A, the lips of the neural folds have not yet closed and fused along the midline. Note the inside positive transepithelial potential (*TEP*; actually transectodermal potential in the embryo). In B, the lips have fused, forming the neural tube. Note the inside of the neural tube was the outside milieu in A, and a TEP is still present; this potential inside the closed tube is negative by about 30–40 mV compared to the abluminal face. This is the TNTP. In C, the output of a microelectrode is shown, referenced to the pond water the embryo was maintained in during electrical measurements. Penetration of the ectoderm produced a positive shift of about

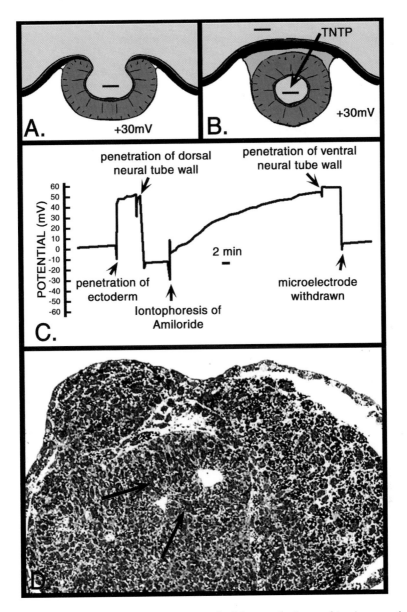

50 mV (the TEP), followed by penetration of the wall of the neural tube, resulting in a negative potential of about 25 mV. Thus, the TNTP in this embryo was ~75 mV across the wall of the neural tube and inside negative. At the point indicated, amiloride was injected into the lumen of the neural tube by iontophoresis. Note the steady collapse of the TNTP to approximately the potential of the TEP. This reveals that the TNTP was produced by the same physiology underlying the generation of the TEP. In D, the results of TNTP collapse (for about 4 h) on development is shown. Note that the integrity of the neural tube is nearly destroyed. An intact portion can be seen in the *upper right*; however, on the *left*, the walls of the tube have disappeared, as these cells have migrated out into the interior of the embryo (*arrows*)

8.2.2
Endogenous Voltages During Neural Tube Formation

Recall that at the end of neurulation, the most dorsal edges (or lips) of the neural folds fuse, forming the neural tube. This ectoderm surrounds the lumen that is filled with fluid, once the outside domain of the embryo (Fig. 17). This inside-out ectoderm still supports a TEP across itself, which would be expected to be positive on the basal side with respect to the apical surface (Fig. 17). After fusion of the neural folds, the apical surface becomes the luminal surface of the neural tube. Thus, the luminal surface of the neural tube is negative with respect to the abluminal surface. This has been directly measured with microelectrodes, which were passed through the overlying ectoderm (first revealing the TEP) and further into the lumen of the neural tube to sample the transneural tube potential (TNTP) (Shi and Borgens 1995). This TNTP in the urodele embryo is ~60–80 mV (inside negative), which results in an electrical field across the wall of the neural tube (a width on the order of 30–50 μm) that can be larger than 1 V/mm (Shi and Borgens 1995). Since the microelectrode tip was advanced into the lumen of the neural tube to measure its TNTP, amiloride and benzamil could subsequently be iontophoresed into the lumen, collapsing the TNTP (Fig. 17). This experiment demonstrated the TNTP to be analogous to the typical amiloride-sensitive TEP of surface ectoderm, as one might expect. Further, it provided an additional means of testing the developmental relevance of the TNTP. Temporary collapse of the TNTP (for ~ 3–4 h at stage 20–21 in the axolotl) produced gross malformation and deletions of developing structure, particularly in the head region of embryos, that were apparent 3–4 days later. In fact, axolotl embryos could continue to develop for several days after such a short manipulation, but without any head at all (Shi and Borgens 1994; Borgens and Shi 1995). Other common malformations included deletions of CNS accessory structures such as the otic, optic, and olfactory placodes and the curious production of two ventricular/cisternal systems in the brain (Metcalf and Borgens 1994; Shi and Borgens 1994; Borgens and Shi 1995).

--➤

Fig. 18A–C. Galvanotropisms in neurons, glia, and muscle. In A–C, the cathodal orientation of neurites extending from individual developing embryonic *Xenopus* neuroblasts are shown. These photographs are over 20 years old and were part of the data from the original work of Laura Hinkle, Ken Robinson, and Colin McCaig (Hinkle et al. 1981). The cells were plated on tissue culture plastic and not on an organic substrate. The more prominent turning behavior towards the cathode is emphasized in the accompanying tracings in A', B', and C'. Within minutes of the time the voltage gradient was imposed across the culture chamber, neurites ceased random growth and made right angle turns directly towards the cathode as shown in A' and C'. Note the perpendicular orientation of myoblasts in the voltage gradient in A. A robust cathodal orientation in many individual *Xenopus* neurons is shown *below*, where the cell bodies of each neuron was superimposed over one another after several serial experiments. To the *left*, the random orientation of neurites is revealed as an approximately equidistant halo of neurites prior to field exposure. On the *right*, a strong orientation of the same neurites towards the cathode is shown after field exposure. Each montage was produced by tracing the course of neurite growth over 5 h, prior to and after exposure to a voltage gradient of 150 mV/mm. Note the marked enhancement of the rate of growth towards the cathode. In most cases, galvanotropisms are observed in response to imposed voltage gradients of 10–500 mV/mm strengths, with the overall vigor of the response dependent upon field strength. The direction of orientation in the

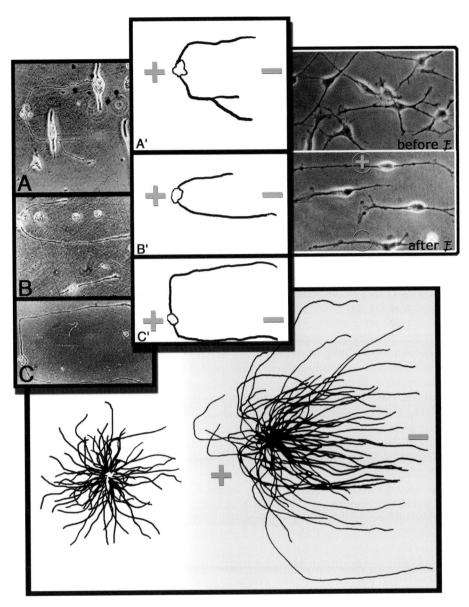

applied field is based on several factors, including the type of substrate and its net charge. In general, neurites grow towards the cathode in physiological magnitudes of electrical fields and on physiological substrates (see text). The two photomicrographs at the *top right* show the responses of cultured GFAP⁺ rat cortical astrocytes to applied voltages. The *upper photograph* shows a population of these cells bearing numerous processes prior to exposure to the electrical field. The *lower photograph* is the same field of view and reveals the typical response of astrocytes to fields on the order of 100–500 mV/mm hours later. Within a few minutes after exposure to the electrical field, astrocytes pull in their many processes, and re-extend, usually two processes, perpendicular to the long axis of the applied voltage, as shown. Curiously, the presence of the field not only provides orientation cues, but also induces a bipolar architecture upon astrocytes in culture (Borgens et al. 1994)

Early evaluation of embryos with TNTP collapse showed that the neural tube did not die (there was no evidence of cell death); rather it disaggregated, appearing to dedifferentiate (Borgens and Shi 1995, Fig. 17D). This notion was supported by the observation that in a surprising proportion of treated embryos (and not saline injected controls), dedifferentiation of all internal structures had occurred, producing pseudoembryos. These animals continued to develop for some days after the TNTP collapse, becoming sickle-shaped in external appearance, similar to normally developing embryos. Closer examination of the histology revealed they were composed of a nearly unbroken expanse of undifferentiated cells (Borgens and Shi 1995). This raised the interesting possibility that the control of external morphogenesis may be mediated in part by the transembryonic currents and voltage gradients, while internal histogenesis may be dependent, in part, on the physiological functioning of developing epithelia syncytia, the rudiments of the organ systems. Furthermore, the anatomical integrity of the epithelium is likely dependent on the proper functioning of ion pumps and channels inserted into its membranes as it develops.

These two electrical controls (transembryonic electrical fields and the TNTP) may be uncoupled from each other by careful electrical manipulation (Shi and Borgens 1995). Currently we are working to reveal the way these physiological controls of development are tied to the better appreciated molecular and genetic controls of morphogenesis using the embryonic limb system, in collaboration with William Scott and Shelia Bell at the Children's Hospital Research Foundation in Cincinnati, Ohio.

It is also tantalizing to speculate that such a large and polarized voltage gradient as the endogenous TNTP may help order developing cells as they differentiate to form the substance of the brain and spinal cord. There are several lines of circumstantial evidence to suggest this may be so. The neurons and glia of the embryonic CNS differentiate from a neuroepithelium, the birth of neurons occurring nearest the luminal face of the neural tube, with their subsequent migration towards the surface. The pathways of pioneer neurites are in part guided by a scaffolding of radial glial cells and their processes, which predates the movement of neurons or their processes. This blueprint is part of classic descriptive studies by Pasco Rakic at Yale University (Rakic 1971a, b).

The magnitude of the TNTP (negative on the inner face with respect to the outer face) would be greatest near the luminal surface, where tight junctions provide the electrical seal for the tube. This region of the largest voltage drop is where neurons are born. Extracellular electrical fields have already been shown to facilitate the survival and the development of neurons from neuroblasts, defined by the enhanced formation of neurites in vitro (Hinkle et al. 1981).

Interestingly, the early dendrites produced by mammalian hippocampal neurons in vitro clearly order themselves toward the cathode of an applied electrical field, while axons project towards the anode (Davenport and McCaig 1993; Rajnicek et al. 1992). The orientation of glial cells and their processes can also be influenced by an extracellular electrical field. In culture, striking perpendicular alignment of GFAP$^+$ astrocytes occurs in response to an imposed voltage gradient orders of magnitude lower than that naturally produced across the neural tube (Borgens et al. 1994; Fig. 18). Furthermore, a very modest shift in the alignment of astrocytes within the adult rat spinal cord in vivo can be induced by an applied gradient of voltage (Moriarty and Borgens 2001). Perhaps this large TNTP: (1) helps promote the survival and differentiation of neurons, (2) helps to orient the processes of radial glia, and (3) provides accessory guidance cues for the subsequent migration and maturation of neurons. Later in the text (Chap. 10, "The Responses of Isolated Nerve Fibers in Culture to Applied DC Voltages", Figs. 18 and 19), I will discuss these cell orientations in response to an extracellular voltage gradient, and the nature of the substrate in establishing this order. Suffice it to say that it is an interesting and testable proposition that the establishment of the amiloride-sensitive TNTP, which occurs at the time of the closure of the neural tube, may be important not only for the integrity of the tube itself (Borgens and Shi 1995), but may confer a general anatomical order upon the early developing cells of the CNS. Experiment number 50 or 60 in my list of things to do is to directly test this notion by using conventional voltage clamp techniques to set the TNTP to a desired magnitude and polarity for a period of hours, and then to determine the effect of this treatment on the architecture of neurons and glia compared to sham-treated control animals.

In summary, steady, polarized DC extracellular voltage gradients are a normal environmental component in the early developing nervous system. Interference with these natural voltages causes predictable anatomical malformations, testifying to their relevance to development.

9 Endogenous Voltages and the Reaction of the Neuron to Injury

Strictly speaking, the preceding analogy of the embryonic ectoderm or the adult integument to a battery is a sound one. The physiology of these structures provides a separation of charge across membrane(s) that can serve as an electromotive force (EMF) driving electric current through cells or across their membranes and/or partitioning macromolecules in their membranes based on their charge as discussed.

It is important to consider the cell membrane as another such battery. It has been known for over 100 years that cells or animals can drive injury currents through themselves. The first man to measure the action potential in nerve, E. DuBois-Reymond was also one of the first physiologists to measure skin wound currents in man by galvanometric techniques (DuBois-Reymond 1860; see also Herlitzka 1910). The famous student of Ramón y Cajal, Rafael Lorenti de Nó measured demarcation potentials in injured nerve with low-impedance galvanometers using surface electrodes. He considered the movement of current and the steady electrical potential as a means to convey information concerning the size and locus of the breach in the membrane to the cell body: *"It is thinkable, therefore, that the continued flow of the demarcation current into the last few millimeters of regenerating nerve is a mechanism by means of which energy is transferred to the regenerating end from points at some distance from it"* (Lorente de Nó 1947, p 459). As it turns out, the ancient means to measure injury currents with low-impedance galvanometers were more informative than modern attempts using high-impedance electrometers. In the former method, a sizable amount of current gained access to the low input resistance meter, and was measured. Thus, the magnitude of the bioelectric potentials in these very old data was conservative, and the polarity correct. In the more modern method using high-impedance multimeters, surface contact electrodes sampled a voltage between them that was dependent on the resistance between them (on the surface of the sample, given by Ohms Law), which can be highly variable. In practice, modern investigators dried the surface of the specimen as a means to elevate this resistance to produce artificially high, but measurable, potential drops. Thus, the magnitude of these bioelectric potentials was unnaturally high, though the polarity of the voltage gradient many times turned out to be correct. Generally, the historical literature of injury to skin suggested the local region of the injury would be positive relative to regions farther away, which, as discussed above, is correct (review Fig. 14).

With regard to surface potentials on exposed peripheral nerves such as measured by Lorente de Nó (1947) and Cowan (1934), the region of injury to the nerve would be negative on the surface with respect to undamaged areas. This is because ionic current is driven into injured axons since they are internally negative with respect to the outside. Being as charitable as one can, injury potential measurements (or demarcation potentials) of the 1950s–1970s were often right for the wrong reasons. It remained an unconvincing literature until the late 1970s when the extracellular vibrating electrode was used to noninvasively evaluate injury currents in nerve fibers and put these issues on sound physiological grounds (reviewed by Borgens 1982).

The first noninvasive direct measurements of electric current entering the breach in single axons were made using reticulospinal axons of the ammocoete lamprey spinal cord by Lionel Jaffe, Melvin Cohen, and myself (Borgens et al. 1980). Transection of the spinal cord in organ culture (with the brain intact) produced currents approaching 500 $\mu A/cm^2$ entering the stump of the amputated cord. Remarkably large peaks (approaching 1 mA/cm^2) were sometimes detected entering the open bore of giant reticulospinal axons when the vibrating electrode was positioned adjacent, but not touching, their cut ends. Indeed, huge ionic currents entered the breach in the axolemma and current flowed through the terminal part of this "cable" in a distal-proximal direction. The associated voltage gradient within the axon due to this flow of current can be many mVs/mm (see Borgens and McCaig 1989) and would be positive at the cut face inside the axon with respect to regions of the cytosol further from the cut end. This voltage is large enough to partition differently colored fluorescent dyes depending on their charge. I have iontophoretically injected both rhodamine (red in color and positively charged) and Lucifer yellow (yellow and negatively charged) into lamprey giant axons using a double-barreled pipette. After crushing the axons, the markers began to separate, Lucifer moving towards the injury and rhodamine moving away from it (unpublished observations; however, see also Cooper et al. 1989). By exchanging and replacing ions in the bathing media, my colleagues and I were able to determine the relative composition of the net injury current entering lamprey giant axons. It largely mirrored the majority ions in the extracellular medium, being mostly a Na^+ (~70%) current, the balance carried by an influx of the cation Ca^{++}. The striking increases in concentration near the cut end – within the cytosol – of these two ions would be catastrophic to the stability of the cytosol, as we discussed in Chap. 2, Sect. 2.2.2, "Secondary Injury". Using the intracellular Ca^{++} probe, Fura II, the increases in terminal Ca^{++} was so great (also measured in severed lamprey giant axons) that it interfered with the ability to precisely measure its concentration, (since it was greater than saturation for Fura II detection (Strautman et al. 1990). Such a high concentration in cytoplasm liquifies the terminal ends of cut axons (see Zelena 1969; Zelena et al. 1968).

The neurobiologist must consider the ionic derangement in nerve cells in response to breaches in the membrane, not as the passive and unimpeded mixing of ions flowing down their concentration gradients, but as a dynamic, metabolically driven event.

10 The Responses of Isolated Nerve Fibers in Culture to Applied DC Voltages

10.1
Historical Pespective

The notion that applied gradients of voltage could provide directional information to growing nerve fibers probably began with the studies of Sven Ingvar in 1920. For the next 60 years (for example, Weiss 1934 to Sisken and Smith 1975) this subdiscipline of neuroscience remained controversial, and a clear unambiguous demonstration that extracellular voltages could indeed direct the growth of nerve fibers was not provided in these earlier reports. This was in part due to the technical inability of the times to precisely measure the magnitude or geometry of applied extracellular fields within culture chambers, and a yet immature understanding of substrate interactions with growing nerve fibers. The most thoughtful and accomplished early investigation was performed by Gordon Marsh and Harold Beams at Iowa State University, the year of my birth, in 1946. The first well-controlled modern demonstration of electrical-field responses by neurites growing out of explanted chick dorsal root ganglia was by Lionel Jaffe and Moo-ming Poo in 1979. This report rendered all previous experiments obsolete. These authors evaluated the historical literature noting:

1. A failure to describe directional responses of growing nerve fibers (neurites) within the imposed electrical field at all (fibers that cannot be identified as being axons or dendrites are referred to as neurites).
2. A failure to use salt bridges to carry current to the culture dish. Earlier attempts inserted metallic electrodes directly into the culture medium, contaminating it with the products of electrolysis.
3. A failure to record the movement of the ganglion (the central cell mass from which nerve fibers were extending). If neurites are attached at their tips to the substrate, and the ganglion moves toward the anode, this would mimic neurite elongation towards the cathode.
4. A failure to record the changes or movement in the organic substrate (such as a plasma clot) upon which the ganglion were growing.
5. A failure to consider the effects of the viscosity of the culture medium in enhancing or detracting from nerve fiber growth responses. This is an important control for the possible formation of chemical gradients within the media that could account for neurite orientation.

An important component of the Jaffe and Poo (1979) experiment was that the polarity of the applied voltage was reversed mid-experiment. The rate of nerve process growth towards the new cathode was then increased, while those nerve fibers facing the new anode were retarded. A slight movement of the cell mass itself in response to the applied voltage was recorded (towards the anode) and subtracted from the cathodal orientation of fibers. Furthermore, Jaffe and Poo varied the viscosity of the medium with methylcellulose to further clarify that the responses of the nerve tissue were due to the imposed voltage and not to the formation of chemical gradients in the culture media produced by the imposed voltage. The results of this first carefully conducted experiment can be summarized as follows:

1. Rates of growth of nerve fibers towards the cathode (negative pole of the applied voltage gradient) were enhanced.
2. Rates of growth towards the anode were reduced.
3. A slight bending towards the cathode by tangential oriented fibers was discerned, though at the level of detection.

All of these responses were dependent on the magnitude of the imposed fields (approximately 1–140 mV/mm), the most marked responses occurring between 70 and 140 mV/mm for periods of observation up to 20 h (Jaffe and Poo 1979).

Experiments such as those of Jaffe and Poo (1979), Sisken and Smith (1975), and Marsh and Beams (1946), were still complicated by the fact that nerve cell masses (ganglion) must be affixed to a substrate in culture to thrive, and when they do thrive, they produce hundreds of processes, which grow out of the central cell mass like hair. This fact complicated evaluation of subtle effects of applied voltages, particularly on the possible direction of growth of individual small nerve processes or their growth cones. Two subsequent landmark reports within 1 year of each other provided further clarification of directional responses by single nerve cell fibers to applied voltages (Hinkle et al. 1981; Patel and Poo 1982). Both of these experiments utilized single, disaggregated nerve cells obtained from embryonic frog nervous system, cultured upon tissue culture plastic and *not* upon an organic substratum (such as a plasma clot, collagen or another organic surface). For the first time, investigators could observe the responses of single cells and their processes in isolation from each other and in the absence of the sometimes confusing interaction of the cell with its substrate.

The data from both Hinkle et al. (1981) and Patel and Poo (1982) can be summarized as follows:

1. Single nerve cell processes react within minutes of exposure to the field (10–100 mV/mm) and grow towards the cathode. They retract away from the anode within hours of exposure. Sometimes the retraction of the nerve process away from the positive pole could lead to complete reabsorption of the fiber into the cell body.
2. Nerve fiber growth towards the cathode can be striking with individual fibers making right angle turns to orientate themselves parallel with the long axis of the voltage gradient (Fig. 18).

3. More single nerve cells began development in culture, that is, producing nerve fibers when exposed to the extracellular voltage gradient than those cultured without it.

4. Moo-ming Poo revealed that the axis of the imposed field could be changed in mid-experiment, specifying a new direction of growth of individual neurites. Poo et al. (1982) also demonstrated that neurites could respond to an inhomogeneous (focally) applied electric field (produced by delivering current to the medium via a microelectrode) in a manner similar to the way they responded to a homogeneously applied field (that is uniformly expressed across the entire culture chamber). In studies of neurotrophic substances, such as NGF, fibers grow "up" the increasing concentration gradient of the factor, the source being the tip of a pipette (Zheng et al. 1994; Ming et al. 1997). Poo discovered that nerves respond to voltage gradients in the same way.

5. Symmetric alternating current (AC) fields do not provide directional cues, unless the polarity of the current pulse in one direction is exaggerated in time or magnitude relative to the other (i.e., an asymmetric AC field). The more asymmetric the waveform, the more directional information provided growing nerves. One can think of this as the more the AC field approaches the characteristic of a DC field (by accentuating the polarity of one pulse at the expense of the other), the better the guidance cues provided to the growing nerve process.

10.2
Galvanotaxis: Rules and Trends

Colin McCaig of the University of Aberdeen was an original member of the team that first used single nerve cells in culture to document their responses to weak applied voltages (Hinkle et al. 1981). He and his colleagues have continued to further elaborate and clarify these seminal observations for the 20 years since. In particular, he has explored the interaction of electric fields and substrate on nerve guidance and the mechanisms of action involved in transducing the extracellular field via the recognized molecular determinants of nerve growth.

To establish a basis for understanding for the reader, I am first going to set some rules and trends that have emerged from 25 years of modern investigation of galvanotaxis. I am doing this with the full knowledge that under some experimental conditions there will be exceptions to these rules, which, as always, further research may clarify or nullify. This is the best any of us can do in science faced with such dynamic complexity. First let us establish these norms.

1. Under physiological conditions and on physiological substrates (see point 5 below), axons will turn towards the cathode (negative pole) of a weak applied voltage gradient (Fig. 18).

2. Anodal facing fibers may turn away, even be reabsorbed into the cell body. Often, they may continue to grow towards the anode but at much reduced rates. For example, *Xenopus* neurites in culture grow toward the cathode at ~30 μm/h, while towards the anode, at ~3–4 μm/h (McCaig 1986).

3. The turning of neurites towards the cathode after the experimenter changes the polarity of the application mid-experiment or of neurites that had emerged from the cell body at approximately right angles to the voltage gradient, is usually accompanied by an approximate threefold increase in their rate of growth.
4. Filopodia are greatest in number and activity on the cathode-facing side of the growth cone preceding a turn in this direction.
5. The net charge on the surface of the substrate that neurites are growing helps determine their overall response to an applied voltage. Thus, field-induced orientation of neurites growing on a laminin surface is similar to the original studies of neurite navigation on falcon tissue culture plastic (also possessing a net negative charge). Poly-L-lysine, a common culture substrate, is positively charged, and supports turning in the opposite direction (towards the anode). This observation was further corroborated by using other plastic surfaces of known charge density (Rajnicek et al. 1998). For example, Plastek M (negatively charged) supported better cathodal orientation of neurites than Plastek C (positively charged).
6. When the adhesiveness of the polylysine substrate was increased, by increasing concentration, greater turning towards the anode occurred.

The dynamic navigation of neurites on plastic substrates in response to an applied electrical field absolutely destroys the skeptic's notion (unsupported by any modern citations that I am aware of) that the imposed voltage gradient is not read by the growth cone, but instead, is influenced by a reorganization of the substrate molecules induced by the voltage (see Jaffe and Nuccitelli 1977).

Mammalian cells in culture respond similarly, in most respects, as frog or chick neurites in the seminal studies. They usually exhibit preferential growth towards the cathode under physiological conditions; however, more recent investigation has revealed important and interesting subtleties.

Rat hippocampal neurons in culture are known to produce neurites that can be identified as becoming either axon or dendrite. Several neurites are formed on an individual cell, but only one of them differentiates as an axon; the remaining neurites become dendrites. Interestingly, the longest of the group becomes the axon. This predisposition can be revealed by cutting the processes to different lengths and then recording their fate (Goslin and Banker 1989). Davenport and McCaig (1993) showed that hippocampal pyramidal neurites destined to become dendrites initially turned towards the cathode of a focally applied electric field. However, more than one-third of this population did not sustain this cathodal orientation. Axons (the longer processes) either did not show a directional response to the applied field, or turned towards the anode.

We have previously considered that the large (up to 1 V/mm) endogenous TNTP of the neural tube might impose:

1. An initial polarity on the directed migration of neurons born near the luminal surface (See Shi and Borgens 1994)
2. An orientation on radial glia that form a template for their growth (see Hatten 1991; Borgens et al. 1995)
3. A polarity on the emerging dendritic field, while at the same time influencing a different axonal projection from the same cell (as in Davenport and McCaig 1993)

This may be true, but such a notion would be unrealistically stretching the inferences of the Davenport and McCaig report. As the authors remark, both the initiation site(s) and the orientation of hippocampal axons from their respective cell bodies in culture were perpendicular to the axis of an applied homogeneous field (Rajnicek et al. 1992; as opposed to the focal ones used in Davenport and McCaig 1993). Microelectrode tips were also placed very near the growth cones, ~20 μm from them. They also discuss the different elongation rates of the neurites, as well as their age in culture, as critical factors when considering these interesting but peculiar responses by hippocampal neurons.

In my opinion, the most important contribution of this unique study is that under controlled conditions, the growth cones of different anatomical classes of nerve fibers from the same cell responded differently to the applied voltage. This proves these kinds of responses are dynamic active choices made by different parts of the same neuron.

10.3
Extracellular Voltages and the Choices Neurons Make

There are many lines of evidence that extracellular voltages integrate with the other types of extrinsic orientation cues and share numerous mechanisms of action with them in playing out the response. One should expect this since in the embryo all of these guidance factors exist with each other and it would be ridiculous to consider their actions as independent and not interrelated.

1. Applied voltages act synergistically with neurotrophic substances to induce greater rates of growth and branching than either factor individually. Neurotrophic substances tested in the presence of applied fields include NGF, BDNF, NT 3, NT 4, and CTNF. Turning and branching behavior induced by the presentation of the applied electric field is sometimes strikingly enhanced by addition of growth factors, and such robust sprouting is usually directed cathodally. McCaig et al. 2000 summarized the results of these studies: (a) certain neurotrophins reduce the threshold in magnitude of the field strength required to redirect neurite growth in culture, (b) neurotrophins increased the numbers of fibers being redirected by the field, (c) neurotrophins produced a bi-modal response in the presence of NT 3. At low field strengths (~10 mV/mm), NT 3 (100 ng/ml) induced anodal turning in embryonic *Xenopus* neurites that would ordinarily orient towards the cathode, which switched to a robust cathodal orientation at higher field strengths, and (d) either the electric field or the neurotrophic factor alone could modify neuronal behavior in vitro, but when tested together, branching indices and rates of growth were statistically significantly greater when they were in combination.
2. Neurites growing along a score in the floor of a plastic culture dish are redirected away from the score when an applied field is placed orthogonal to it. The re-established direction of growth is towards the cathode of the applied electrical field. Thus, contact guidance cues can be overridden by applied voltages (McCaig 1986; Fig. 19). This is not true for very adhesive substrates such as laminin. When a laminin track is placed at right angles and in the pathway of cathodally directed neurites (<100 mV/mm), only approximately one-third of the nerve fibers will

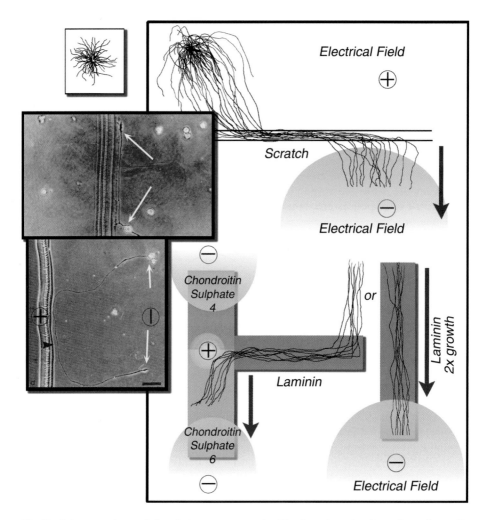

Fig. 19. Galvanotropism and the choices neurons make. Neurite orientation is random when cells are cultured on tissue culture plastic in the absence of orientational cues. The photomicrographs on the *left* show that neurites will follow a score in the plastic substrate by contact guidance mechanisms. At the *bottom* of the *top photograph* the *arrow* points to the cell body, and at the *top*, another *arrow* points to the growth cone as it extends upwards along the score. The *lower* photograph shows a neurite turning away from the score when provided another orientation cue, the cathode of an applied voltage gradient. The cell body is at the *top*, and the growth cone at the *bottom* of the photograph. The *dark arrowhead* indicates the point when a voltage gradient was imposed across the chamber at right angles to the score as indicated. At physiological field strengths, neurons prefer to follow voltage-mediated cues rather than contact guidance cues. In the drawings to the *right*, the choices neurites make when provided simultaneous guidance cues are represented. At the *top*, neurites are extending along a scratch by contact guidance, until presented a choice, and then turn away from the score and towards the negative pole of an extracellular voltage gradient (in the direction of the *red arrow*). These neurites will increase their rate of growth (approximately two to three times) if they are presented a laminin pathway, extending in the same direction as the long axis of the electrical field shown at the *far right*. However, if the growing neurites intercept a laminin pathway, which extends orthogonal to their direction of growth within the electrical field, they will turn away

88

continue in a cathodal direction; the bulk will turn to orient on the laminin surface (Fig. 19). If neurites were extending on a 25-μm-wide track, a similar magnitude of DC field was unable to induce neurites to leave this pathway (Britland and McCaig 1996).

3. Growing neurites can also interpret cues presented by voltage gradients simultaneous with those presented by membrane-bound molecular guidance cues. Chondroitin sulfate proteoglycans are normal components of the ECM and have well-described abilities to attract nerve growth in some cases, or repulse nerve growth in others (Snow et al. 1990, 1991; Snow and Letourneau 1992). When the orientation of neurites in culture was established by an imposed voltage gradient (50–200 mV/mm), exposure to chondroitin 4 sulfate inhibited cathodal orientation, while chondroitin 6 sulfate enhanced growth towards the cathode (Fig. 19). Furthermore, this effect was established to be due to the glycosaminoglycan side chains for each macromolecule and not dependent on the protein core (Erskine and McCaig 1997).

4. The cell responses to both ECMs and CAMs are mediated by macromolecules floating in the plasmalemma (e.g., integrins and/or receptors) and so too are applied voltages. Over 2 decades ago, Moo-ming Poo showed that the orientational cues provided by imposed voltage gradients could be blocked by the addition of the lectin Concanavalin A (ConA) to the media. ConA both binds to and reduces the mobility of receptors spanning the membrane. This result suggested early on that receptors, and likely their redistribution within the plane of the membrane, mediate galvanotaxis.

5. The mechanisms of action underlying the orientation/reorientation of neurons and their processes in response to molecular growth factors is known to involve second messenger systems and likely a regulated entry of Ca^{++} into regions of extension of the neuritic process, as do the responses of neurons to electrical fields. For example, the adenyl cyclase stimulant, forskolin, induces a marked increase in the rate of elongation of neurites, as does a physiological electrical field. When these two factors are combined in one experiment, their action is additive (as long as the concentration of forskolin is held 50 μM). Calcium's role has been dis-

---

from the latter cue and grow instead along the laminin path. In this experimental situation, the laminin trumps the electrical field, just as the field trumps contact guidance along irregularities in terrain. To the *left* in this odyssey, fibers are again presented an electrical field as a cue simultaneous with a different organic substrate of proteoglycans. An additive effect on turning and growth rate is observed towards chondroitin 6 sulfate and away from chondroitin 4 sulfate, even in the presence of a distally negative voltage gradient. This series of investigations by Colin McCaig, Ann Rajnicek and their colleagues at the University of Aberdeen Medical School in Scotland clearly demonstrates that growth cones can interpret several types of guidance cues simultaneously, and make choices based on these. The presence of an extracellular voltage gradient of a physiological magnitude is one of these naturally occurring guidance factors. This cue can supersede others, and be superseded by still others. Most importantly, neurites can sum these cues to respond more vigorously than to either cue independently. This is the same interpretative power possessed by growing neurites and revealed in the presence of soluble neurotrophic factors in addition to extracellular electrical fields (see text)

cussed above, and will be dealt with again in a later discussion in the next chapter.

Numerous receptors and receptor complexes have been established to move freely in the plane of the membrane in an imposed electric field, accumulating in the local membrane at one pole of the cell or the other (see Jaffe 1977; Poo 1981; McLaughlin and Poo 1981; Young and Poo 1983; Linliu et al. 1984; McClosky and Poo 1984). Lateral electrophoresis and electro-osmosis (McClaughlin and Poo 1981) provides the physical basis for membrane receptor redistribution. Numerous membrane-spanning receptors are now known to reversibly distribute in physiological extracellular electric fields. Four of the first studied examples include: ConA receptors (Poo and Robinson 1977), acetylcholine (ACh) receptors (Orida and Poo 1978); basophilic leukemia Fc receptors (McClosky et al. 1984), and epidermal growth factor receptors (Giugni et al. 1987). Membrane spanning macromolecules that bind the plant lectin ConA include both the conductance channel for ACh and its receptors (Orida and Poo 1982). Pretreatment of neurons with ConA prior to imposition of the electrical field, crosslinks and immobilizes these receptors so that they cannot move within the membrane when exposed to a gradient of voltage, producing a failure in the normal cathodal orientation of the neurites (Patel and Poo 1982). If we connect these dots with recent reports revealing that ACh can act as a neurotrophic factor, intriguing possibilities begin to emerge.

The dots are:

1. Under physiological conditions, ACh receptors accumulate on the cathodal facing membranes of neurites, the pole to which the growth cone will turn when in physiological conditions.
2. Redistribution of ACh receptors in that imposed electrical field can be blocked by ConA, which also destroys the orientational response.
3. ACh can also beckon neurites to grow towards a diffusing source of the neurotransmitter mediated by an asymmetric increase in intracellular Ca^{++} (Zheng et al. 1996).
4. Receptor-mediated increases in Ca^{++} within growth cones can be blocked by several voltage-sensitive channel blockers, which as well inhibits their orientation and growth in the imposed electrical field.
5. Field-induced turning behavior can also be inhibited by the ACh receptor antagonist *d*-tubocurarine (Erskine and McCaig 1995; Stewart et al. 1995). McCaig has connected some of these dots in McCaig et al. 2000, also instructing that BDNF and NT 3 also induce the release of ACh at the neuromuscular junction.

I cannot *yet* say it is clear that many of the mechanisms underlying voltage-mediated guidance and branching in nerves share substantial mechanisms of action with similar actions of the ECM and chemical growth factors. However, this issue is clearing up rapidly, and an affirmative answer I believe is already apparent.

11 Enhancing Spinal Cord Regeneration In Situ with Applied Electric Fields

11.1
The Control of Regeneration of Nerve Fibers in the Fish Spinal Cord by Applied Electric Fields

The first unambiguous demonstration of enhanced spinal cord nerve regeneration in the living animal was carried out in a primitive fish, the ammocoete larvae of the lamprey (Borgens et al. 1981). This investigation utilized the special characteristics of the lamprey brain and spinal cord. In this animal, individually identifiable giant nerve cells in the brain (Müller and Mauthner cells) give rise to descending nerve fibers that are also identifiable in the spinal cord as part of the descending reticulospinal system (Rovainen 1967, 1974). Since the lamprey is an Agnathan, a primitive cartilaginous fish, there is no bony vertebral column surrounding and protecting the spinal cord: the cord and brain is easy for the investigator to surgically expose. Therefore, the fish system provides some of the same advantages as nerve fibers in culture where the investigator can describe the regeneration or growth of specific individual and identifiable nerve cells. The cell bodies of lamprey reticulospinal neurons are giant (~100 μm in diameter) and so are their spinal cord axons (~30 μm), making them easy to fill with intracellular dyes from a micropipette and to identify at any location within the brain and spinal cord (Wood and Cohen 1979; Borgens 1981) (Fig. 20).

At Yale University in the late 1970s, Melvin Cohen, Ernesto Roederer, and I imposed distally negative, weak voltage gradients across completely transected lamprey spinal cords for approximately 5–7 days using minute salt bridges (nonmetallic wick electrodes). Thus, the voltage gradient was applied along the spinal cord without electrode product contamination produced by metallic electrodes. The regulated current source was external to each small finger bowl where the larvae were maintained suspended in aerated aquarium water by the electrodes. They were released to the aquarium after the electrodes were withdrawn from the body. The cathode was located caudal (towards the tail) to the site where the spinal cord was cut into two segments, the anode rostral to the plane of transection. In this way, descending nerve processes would be influenced to grow since they would be facing the negative pole of the imposed electric field. It should be pointed out that the lamprey spinal cord axons regenerate naturally. First, they die back away from the plane of transection, and then begin to form growth cones at their tips and regenerate. Typically, at 13–15 C, it takes about 120–150 days for descending reticulospinal fibers to regenerate

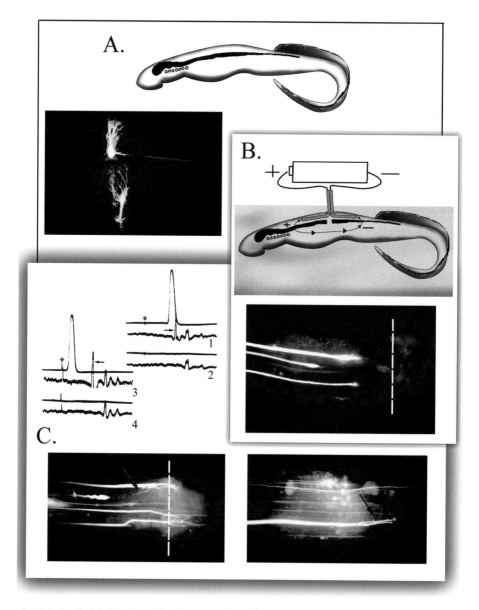

Fig. 20A–C. Electrical field-mediated regeneration of lamprey spinal axons. In **A**, the amocoete lamprey is shown (averaging about 5 cm in length) and the orientation of giant cells in the third ventricle of the brain (*inset*). A Mauthner cell, with its decussating axon, and a Müller cell are shown after intracellular filling with Lucifer yellow, projecting axons out of the hindbrain into the spinal cord. There are 18 such giant cells in the larval lamprey, each individually identifiable. In **B**, a schematic of an electrical circuit is shown, the stimulator apparatus was placed above individual finger bowls of aerated water containing the larvae. Small-diameter wick electrodes were surgically located on either side of a complete transection of the spinal cord. The negative electrode was located caudal to the projection of these descending reticulospinal axons. Approximately 10 µA of total current was applied, producing an estimated field strength of 10 mV/mm. The *photomicrograph* immediately *be*

and cross the transection plane. Our experiment was terminated at about 50 days after transection, a time when control fibers in sham-treated animals would not have reached the site of the lesion. The imposed electrical field increased the rate of regeneration by threefold, inducing fibers to cross the lesion and to make connection in the caudal segment of cord within this time (Borgens et al. 1981) (Fig. 20). The applied voltage approximately quadrupled the amount of branching of regenerating fibers as well as enhancing their rate of growth. Furthermore, simultaneous intracellular and extracellular recording of nerve fiber impulses (single and compound action potentials) revealed that electrically induced regenerating nerve fibers were capable of carrying nerve impulses across the transection plane to target cells in the isolated caudal segment of spinal cord (Borgens et al. 1981) (Fig. 20). For the first time this experiment clearly demonstrated that a weak voltage gradient could enhance functional spinal cord nerve fiber regeneration in vivo.

Several other studies clarified these responses and provided insight into the mechanisms of action in the enhancement of regeneration of spinal cord nerves in this fish model system. Two years following this report, Roederer et al. (1983) compared the

◄───

low the drawing shows the terminal ends of three regenerating reticulospinal axons projecting near, but not through the plane of transection approximately 55 days after surgery. The original plane of transection is shown by the *hatched line* (note the parenchyma was not completely mended, or perhaps separated slightly during handling of the sample). *Below this photograph,* another control cord shows numerous filled axons of different calibers, the largest of which terminates in three regenerating branches (*arrow*). The plane of transection is to the *right* and out of the photographic field. In only a few cases did regenerating giant fibers die back, and then regenerate to enter and cross the lesion by fewer than 60 days after transection at about 15–16°C in sham-treated larvae. At the *bottom left,* an electrical field-treated spinal cord is shown; three of the four Lucifer filled giant fibers have regenerated into the scar and crossed the plane of transection branching numerous times at 59 days after transection. Sometimes the regenerating branches were confused by this terrain and turn back to grow towards the brain (*blue arrow*). The proportion of such fibers that traversed the lesion were statistically significantly greater than sham-treated cords. Recording microelectrodes were filled with Lucifer yellow so that a single identifiable axon that had regenerated through the lesion *and* conducted action potentials (*APs*) across the lesion could be identified. This was accomplished by comparing simultaneously recorded extracellular and intracellular recordings. In **C,** two sets of two pairs of such recordings are shown. In each pair the extracellular record is below the intracellular record. One pair of bipolar extracellular electrodes was placed on the spinal cord caudal to the lesion and stimulation was applied to the hindbrain with a second pair (stimulus artifact marked with an *asterisk*). The extracellular electrode then recorded the numerous action potentials traveling through the lesion associated with regenerating axons. The intracellular microelectrode was inserted into a single identified giant axon and recorded its individual action potential in response to this stimulation. After a series of recordings, the dye was iontophoresed into this axon to mark it. In the pair of recordings marked *1,* the *arrow* points to an extracellular AP in the extracellular record associated with an intracellular recorded AP above it. A subthreshold stimulation eliminated these APs from both records in *2.* Note that other extracellular APs are still recorded. The pair of electrical records in *3* is also an above-threshold stimulation for the axon of interest, and in *4,* a below-threshold stimulation, again identifying a single axon from the extracellular record. Records *3* and *4* were recorded from the same spinal cord as in *1* and *2,* only the stimulation was applied caudal to the lesion, and the APs recorded at the hindbrain (antidromic stimulation). Subsequent labeling confirmed that axons crossing the lesion were functional. (This figure summarizes experiments in Borgens et al. 1981, courtesy of the journal *Science* with permission)

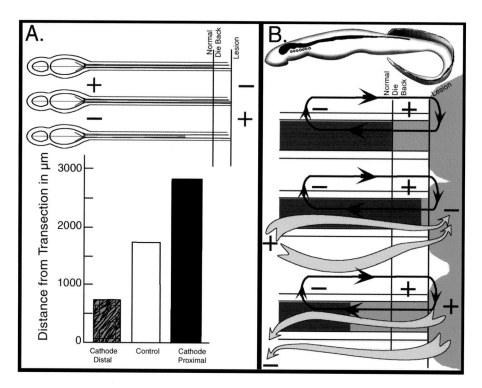

Fig. 21A, B. Voltage-mediated modification of retrograde degeneration in lamprey giant axons. The icons at the *top* in **A** and **B** show the orientation of the CNS used in all the accompanying drawings. In this series of experiments (Roederer et al. 1983), an extracellular voltage was imposed across transected lamprey spinal cord in situ using the same methods as in Borgens et al. 1981 (Fig. 20). The extent of retrograde degeneration from the plane of transection was determined by intracellular labeling of identified descending giant reticulospinal axons. In **A**, the *top drawing* of the lamprey CNS shows the approximate level of axonal die-back in control animals relative to the level of transection. The *second drawing* shows the marked reduction of die-back in distally negative imposed voltage gradients. The *third drawing* shows the effect of the reversed polarity of application, a distally positive imposed field, where the distance of retrograde degeneration was enhanced. The graph is redrawn from that report, showing the mean distance of die-back. To make sense of the next series of drawings in **B**, recall that the direction of current flow is defined as being in the direction that positive charge moves. The drawings on the *right* summarize the experiments of Alan Strautman and colleagues (1991). Similar electrical fields were imposed across lamprey CNS with transected spinal cords. The extent and concentration of Ca^{++} penetration into the cut ends of the proximal segments of giant axons was determined by Fura II detection techniques. Note that a distally negative voltage gradient reduces the net Ca^{++} influx (shown as a *blue* medium) into severed giant axons (shown in *red*), while the opposite polarity enhances Ca^{++} entry. It is believed that the amount of retrograde degeneration of the terminal ends of these axons is reduced in the distally negative electrical field because the direction of the imposed current flow (*yellow*) penetrating the ends of the injured axons would be opposite in direction to the endogenous current (diagrammed in *black*) entering the axon, partly carried by Ca^{++} ions. Said another way, the bucking voltage produced within the end of the damaged axons by the imposed field would tend to repel cations such as Ca^{++} from entering. The opposite polarity of an imposed electrical field would result in the opposite response, enhancing the flow of current into the ends of the cut axons carried in part by cations such as Ca^{++}. It is the destructive effects of Ca^{++} on cytoplasm that lies at the root of retrograde degeneration, and the use of an appropriately oriented electrical field (cathode distal to the cut ends) will both inhibit die-back and promote regeneration and branching of the proximal segment of axon

94

total amount of retrograde degeneration of these same fibers after exposure to a similar electric field in vivo. They found that fibers facing the anode degenerated even further, which bring their cut ends closer to the brain than sham-treated control fibers. Distally negative electric fields (cathodes caudal to the injury) statistically reduced the distance that giant axons died back compared to sham-treated animals (Fig. 21).

This demonstration of a strictly polarized response to an applied DC electric field led Strautman et al. (1990) to further dissect the basis for it. They filled lamprey giant axons with the fluorescent probe for intracellular Ca^{++}, Fura II, and used image intensification techniques to determine the Ca^{++} concentration gradients inside the fibers. They determined that distally positive fields increased the concentration of Ca^{++} entering the cut tips of lamprey spinal cord axons, while the reverse polarity (distally negative fields) strikingly reduced the concentration of Ca^{++} at the injured tip compared to control or sham-treated spinal cords (Strautman et al. 1990). If you take this report along with Roederer et al. 1993, a clear mechanism of action for the inhibition of retrograde degeneration of axons is revealed. Extracellular electric fields reduce or enhance retrograde axonal degeneration and the dissolution of the axonal cytoarchitecture by a direct effect on bucking the endogenous Ca^{++} current entering the cut end or enhancing it, respectively (Fig. 21).

11.2
The Anatomy of Regeneration of Spinal Cord Nerve Fibers in the Laboratory Rat and Guinea Pig

While there have many claims of induced nerve regeneration within the mammalian spinal cord for over 100 years, it has been difficult to determine the credibility of these reports since peripheral nerves can regenerate and often gain access into spinal lesions when the blood–brain barrier is compromised and the tough covering of the cord (the dura) is lacerated (Frisen et al. 1993; Beattie et al. 1997). Furthermore, as emphasized earlier, very few investigations have employed an indwelling marker to reveal the exact plane of injury or transection several months prior to sacrifice of the animal for histology. Our 1986 investigation demonstrating that applied electric fields could induce regeneration of CNS nerve fibers in hemisected mammalian spinal cords employed an indwelling marker device to clearly reveal the original plane of transection (Fig. 22). Regenerating nerve fibers of spinal cord origin were intracellularly marked with both large-molecular-weight dye molecules, HRP, (Borgens 1986b, 1990) and later with small-molecular-weight fluorescent dextrans, conjugated with rhodamine or FITC, (Borgens and Bohnert 1997). Electrical fields were imposed using a completely implantable current-regulated DC stimulator and in early studies, nonmetallic "wick" electrodes (Borgens et al. 1986b, 1990).

Electric fields on the order of approximately 400 μV/mm were imposed across adult guinea pig spinal cord for about 3 weeks, the magnitude of the voltage gradient measured using a quadripole arrangement. In this method, one pair of electrodes was used to pass the current, and one pair (inserted within spinal cord parenchyma) to measure the field strength (Borgens et al. 1990). The negative electrode was placed rostral to the transection plane in all of these experiments, as only the long ascend-

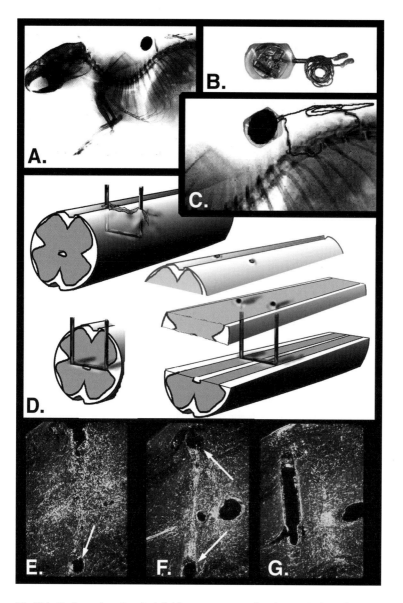

Fig. 22A–G. Imposing electrical fields over transected guinea spinal cord in situ and marking the lesion. In **A**, a radiograph of the guinea pig shows the placement of a miniature DC stimulator (**B**) beneath the fat pad of the animal's back, and the routing of the electrodes to the vertebral column (**C**). In **C**, the stimulator and electrodes in the X-ray is colored by the artist to be more visible. Note that the ends of the electrodes are tied to paravertebral musculature of the spine, and do not enter the canal or touch the spinal cord. The drawings in **D** show the placement of a U-shaped tantalum marker within a dorsal hemisection of the spinal cord. The hemisection of the spinal cord was made with a laboratory-fabricated cutting device and the marker inserted into it. After the cord was fixed and dissected from the animal, a careful clip of the lower corner of the marker allowed it to be withdrawn from the tissues in two pieces, leaving a characteristic pattern of holes in the spinal cord,

ing sensory nerve tracts within the spinal cord were evaluated histologically due to the ease of labeling the dorsal and lateral white matter of the spinal cord.

The results of all studies where voltage gradients were imposed across hemisections of large adult guinea pig spinal cord can be summarized as follows:

1. Sham-treated animals did not reveal evidence of axonal regeneration within labeled spinal cord nerve tracts. Characteristically these fibers, and their collective tracts, die back for distances of about 100–300 μm (sometimes more) from the plane of transection (Fig. 23). Labeled terminals of such static fibers were rarely detected projecting into the scar that had formed at the lesion by 3 months of evaluation after injury, and never crossed the plane of transection. Since intracellular labels were applied at least two vertebral segments (or more) from the lesion, the complicating presence of peripheral axons gaining entrance to the region of the lesion from spinal roots was reduced or eliminated since these roots were not labeled (Borgens and Bohnert 1997).

2. In current-treated cords in the first studies (Borgens et al. 1986b, 1990), a few labeled axons could be traced around the lateral margins of the lesion, through undamaged spinal cord, into the rostral segment. Though labeled regenerating fibers were *very* few in number in any one spinal cord, the numbers of regenerating spinal cords that were current-treated compared to nonregenerating sham-treated cords, was statistically significant (Borgens et al. 1986b, 1990). These regenerating fibers could be traced within the plane of longitudinal sections to and around the lesion. There was no evidence of branching nerve fibers (collateral sprouting) in the long tracts of the caudal segment of cord. Traced axons were singular extensions of axons of the severed dorsal columns and dorsolateral ascending columns. Further studies employed more sensitive low-molecular-weight intracellular labels (rhodamine dextrans). Laser confocal microscopy provided more detail of electrically induced regeneration of nerve fibers in the adult guinea pig-labeled fibers in spinal cords. These studies revealed regenerating nerve fibers not only grew around the margins of the spinal cord lesion, but also projected through the fi-

---

which was then serially sectioned on a rotary microtome. Darkfield photomicrographs, showing descending levels of longitudinal sections of guinea pig spinal cord from a dorsal plane (E) to a ventral plane (G), reveal these holes. In E, the *arrow* points to a clean hole; the upper one tore slightly through the tissue during preparation. In F, the *arrows* show two clean marker holes in a central plane of section, this one just dorsal to the central canal. Note the dorsal aspect of a large CSF-filled syrinx, caudal to the lesion, in this view. In G, a ventral plane of section, below the central canal, reveals the perpendicular-oriented marker hole produced by its base. A slight modification of these procedures also allows the plane of section in a right or left lateral hemisection to be marked. Any longitudinally oriented labeled axon crossing the plane between the holes would have regenerated through the plane of transection. Labeled axons projecting around the holes would have projected to the opposite segment through minimally damaged or undamaged white matter. The distance that axons died back or regenerated relative to the plane of transection was indexed by scribing a line between the holes with a straight edge on working photomicrographs. This effectively revealed the plane of the cut, independent of how large a scar might have formed, how disrupted the tissue was, or the number of months after injury the animal was sacrificed

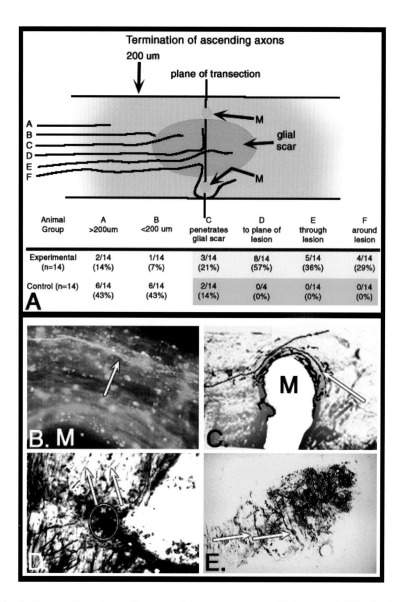

Fig. 23A–E. Regeneration of ascending axons in response to an applied electrical field. The drawing and table summarize the results of experiments where a distally negative voltage gradient was imposed across dorsal hemisections of the guinea pig spinal cord, and the position of the terminal ends of intracellular labeled axons as determined by a marker device to index the plane of transection (see Fig. 22). The negative electrode was placed rostral to the transection to facilitate regeneration of ascending spinal cord axons (mainly in the dorsal columns and ascending lateral tracts). In the drawing, *M* represents marker holes, as in Fig. 22, and the position of various axons in the study is shown by fiber icons **A–F**. Note the position of the 200 μm *arrow* caudal to the plane of transection. Very few fibers penetrated the caudal portion of the glial scar in sham-treated animals (implanted with inoperative stimulators), while in electrically treated animals, fibers projected through and around the lesion. In **B**, the terminal branching of a fluorescently labeled axon is shown (*arrow*).

broglial scar tissue that formed at the site of hemisection (Borgens and Bohnert 1997) (Fig. 23).

11.3
Guiding Spinal Cord Axons into Rubber Tubes with Applied Voltages

In our series of labeling studies, only a very small subpopulation of nerve fibers within the white matter that could potentially respond to the applied voltage (axons numbering in the thousands) were marked by dye injection. These numbers were further reduced because only a small population of labeled fibers retained enough dye to be visualized at the level of the lesion. Our initial claims of spinal axon regeneration in response to applied fields were correct given the tracing methods, the use of markers for the plane of transection, matched controls, and blinded evaluation. On the other hand, a feeble reaction to these results was revealed by our colleagues since regenerating large caliber axons, especially those that were labeled to their terminal ending, were disappointingly few in number. It was also disappointing that we were unable to investigate the ability of the applied voltage gradient to *orient* axonal growth in vivo because so few labeled fibers were available for study.

I used a different experimental approach to determine how robust electrically induced regeneration might be, and if the applied voltage gradient could also direct the regeneration of nerve fibers in the guinea pig spinal cord. In this experiment, the uninsulated portion of a tiny, Teflon-coated cathodal wire (40-gauge multistrand) was inserted into the center of a hollow 6×1-mm-long silicone rubber tube. The tube was surgically implanted into the dorsal half of large adult guinea pig spinal cords

◀──

This individual axon was traced for over 1 cm within thick longitudinal sections of spinal cord to turn and grow around the marker hole in close association with the fibrous scar on the caudal side (*M*, marker hole). In C, the *arrow* points to the terminal end of an HRP-labeled axon that was similarly traced from white matter tracts in the caudal segment of cord, around the transection and through undamaged white matter. Another fiber strays off towards the pial surface just past the level of transection. The artist enhanced these fibers so they could be seen in this photomicrograph reduced in size. The original photomicrographs can be found in Borgens et al. 1990. In B and C, rostral is to the *right*. A reconstructed series of serial 1-μm-thick confocal slices of an electrically treated guinea pig is shown in D. The orientation is caudal to the *bottom*, rostral towards the *top*. The edge of a marker hole can be seen with a thick band of scar tissue projecting from it to the cord's surface. *Arrows* point to labeled axons in the distal segment of cord. Branching and medially projecting fibers are more easily seen in the proximal segment. These fibers were traced from labeled white matter tracts, which were injected two vertebral segments caudal to this confocal image. The *circle* encloses a region of scar tissue shown in E. In E, deletion of multiple confocal images that were comprised of mainly scar tissue cells (and not fibers) allowed these few axons (*arrows*) to be visualized crossing through the scar to the rostral segment (from Borgens and Bohnert 1997). The lack of similar trajectories of fibers in control cords, the longitudinal tracing of individual axons from the site of application of intracellular labels, and the complete absence of dorsal root labeling in all cords revealed these fibers to be of CNS origin. A shortcoming of this series of studies was the small number of such examples found in electrical field-treated animals (see text and Fig. 24)

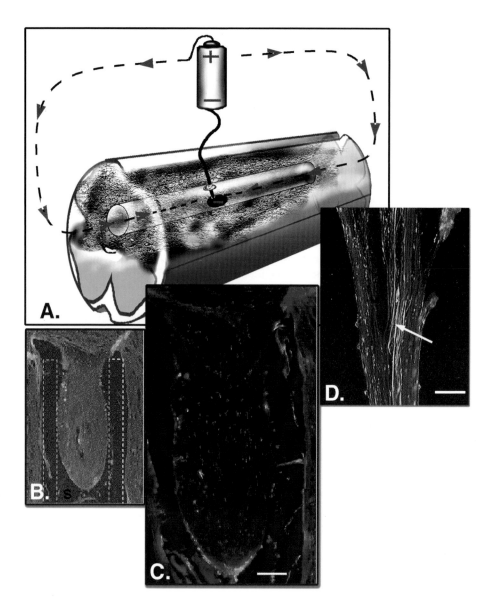

Fig. 24A–D. Growing spinal cord axons into tubes using electrical fields. The drawing in **A** shows the experimental setup from Borgens 1999. A 6×1-mm hollow silastic tube was surgically inserted into the dorsal half of large adult guinea pig spinal cords. This surgery caused significant damage to the cord, severing numerous ascending and descending tracts in the dorsal cord. Prior to implantation, a small silastic insulated electrode wire was inserted into the center of the tube, through a hole, and this hole sealed with silastic glue. The electrode was connected to the negative pole of a small DC stimulator surgically implanted beneath the skin and fat pad of the animal's back. The anodal electrode was left in place at this location. In the animal this created an electrical circuit where current entered each end of the tube as shown. Sham-treated controls were treated identically, except that the stimulator was inoperative. In **B**, a low-power photomicrograph of a longitudinal section of the end of a tube showing the plug of scar tissue that formed inside the mouth of each tube at each

(Fig. 24). The implantation surgery was very destructive to the cord, transecting both ascending and descending dorsal white matter tracts revealed by phalanxes of labeled terminal clubs. Significant gray matter was destroyed as well (Borgens 1999).

This negative electrode was connected to a miniature current-regulated DC stimulator located beneath the skin of the animal's neck, the anode located in the local musculature of the back. With this arrangement, current would be pulled into each end of the hollow silastic tube to complete the circuit (Fig. 24). With the cathode inside, spinal cord axons would be expected to grow up to and into the tube. Since normally large myelinated nerve fibers do not regenerate in the adult guinea pig spinal cord, they could only gain access to the tube by growing there. These active implants were compared to a sham-treated group of animals that contained identical implants; only the voltage sources were internally short circuited and did not deliver current. In all animals, scar tissue formed within the open bore of the tube at both ends, looking like a cork in a wine bottle (Fig. 24). In electrically active implants, the scar tissue plugs that pushed inside the bore of the tube were filled with tangles of regenerating nerve fibers by 2 months after surgery. This time there were so many responding axons, they could not be counted. In control tubes, fibers within the scar plug were very rare. Out of a total of 28 tube ends evaluated in 16 control animals, only 4 axons of unknown origin were detected (Borgens 1999).

To precisely determine the origin of some of the fibers that had regenerated into the tube in electrically treated animals, a retrograde labeling procedure was used. Before the sacrifice of the animals, the top of the silastic tube, where the wire had been glued in place, was exposed surgically, the electrode pulled out of its hole, and a few crystals of rhodamine dye inserted through this hole into the tube. The hole was then sealed with glue. The crystals dissolved in the fluids inside the silastic tube, retrogradely labeling the nerve fibers projecting into it. This labeling procedure proved that of the fibers regenerating into electrically active tubes, some were derived from neurons in nearby intact gray matter. Other retrogradely labeled axons were traced back to the long columns of axons of white matter. The importance of this single study was that it provided formal proof that a very weak imposed electrical field (approximately ≤ 100 μV/mm) can: (1) initiate robust regeneration of nerves within the adult mammalian spinal cord, and (2) such regenerating fibers can be guided by the gradient of voltage to the cathodal (or negative) pole of the applied electrical field (Borgens 1999).

◀——————————————————————————————

end. The approximately 20 μm thick strips of the sectioned walls of the silastic tube were usually lost from the sections during histological processing, but are drawn in with the *hatched lines*. S marks the space within the center of the tube not filled with scar tissue. In C, a fluorescent photomicrograph of this same area shows that anterograde-labeled axons from nearby white matter tracts had not penetrated the scar plug of this sham-treated control tube. In D, the results of an active electrical implant is shown. The scar plug is filled with labeled axons, so many in whorls and tangles that they could not be counted. The shape of the scar plugs was also different in functioning electrical implants. They were more tapered and narrow than the fat and blunt plugs that formed in the control tubes. This suggested that the electrical field affected the reorganization of the nonneuronal cells that filled the ends of the tubes (refer to astrocyte orientations in Fig. 18). (Photomicrographs courtesy of the journal Neuroscience)

11.4
Anatomical Responses to Applied Voltages
by Nonneuronal Cells Important to Spinal Cord Injury:
The Macrophage

Macrophages have been reported to migrate preferentially towards the anode of an applied voltage in culture (Orida and Feldman 1982). Actually, a careful reading of this report does not reveal a true galvanotaxis of macrophages over distance, but the heightened activity of pseudopodial extensions on one side of the phagocyte in a polarized gradient of voltage. Anyway, one could suggest that an applied voltage in situ might induce a migration of macrophages away from the lesion towards one or both electrodes, which are surgically located outside of the vertebral column in rats and guinea pigs. If this electrically enhanced migration depleted the lesion of these phagocytic cells, then this could theoretically contribute to functional recovery through a reduction in the secondary injury cascade. This notion was tested using standardized compression injury to the guinea pig spinal cord and marking activated macrophages within the injury zone with a specific immunocytochemical marker, the monoclonal antibody ED 1 (Damoiseaux 1994). The cells were later counted using a computer-managed morphometry system that did not involve interaction of the investigator with the counting of cells (Moriarty and Borgens 1999). It was learned that the applied voltage (imposed upon the cord by a implantable stimulator system as in the other studies described above) did not influence the density of these cells in the lesion (Moriarty et al. 1999). Thus, if the applied field does exert an effect on CNS repair through an action on the macrophage, it must be on a very subtle, and yet undetected, level.

11.4.1
The Astrocyte

I have already discussed the role of astrocytes in CNS wounds in Chap. 3, Sect. 3.1.1, "Other Inhibitors." As reviewed earlier, it has long been believed that this mat of cells presents some form of a barrier to nerve regeneration and functional recovery in the mammalian spinal cord. Further as discussed, in some vertebrates that regenerate their spinal cord nerves, glial cells are not as plentiful or as disorganized and actually form channels or tubes through which nerve fibers grow to reach the other side of the injury (Singer et al. 1954, reviewed by Chernoff 1995). If the applied voltage could reduce the density of astrocytes multiplying at the spinal cord injury site, it would likely produce a more favorable environment for spinal cord regeneration and eventual functional recovery. This was the point of using enzyme treatments or pyromen administration in early studies of SCI. Furthermore, if the applied field could somehow align astrocytes in a particular way, this might also create conditions more favorable for axonal regeneration within the mammalian cord, as suggested by the observations of spinal cord regeneration in fish and amphibians where this occurs naturally. We had earlier determined that rat cortical astrocytes and their processes were especially sensitive to applied extracellular voltages when tested in vitro. They withdraw their processes shortly after exposure to voltage gradients of 100–500 mV/

mm, and subsequently re-extend them perpendicular to the field as a bipolar cell. Furthermore, astrocytes organize an axis of symmetry within hours of exposure to extracellular electric fields. At higher field strengths, 100% of the population was oriented perpendicular to the axis of the imposed voltage gradient (Borgens et al. 1994) (Fig. 18).

This dramatic change in orientation was difficult to determine in vivo, however. Recently, Loren Moriarty and Borgens (2001) have applied voltages over acute penetrating injury to adult rat spinal cord. This application, strikingly, and statistically significantly, reduced the number of astrocytes forming around the puncture wound. The field also reduced the numbers of astrocytes bearing long cell processes compared to sham-treated controls. Inexplicably, only a modest (≤10%) shift in the preferential orientation of astrocytes was detected in response to the imposed electrical field, and in only undamaged white matter. Astrocytes usually align their long axis parallel with the spinal cord (see Davies et al. 1999 for striking examples). We would have guessed that changes in astrocyte orientation would occur in the loosely organized stroma of the scar, and less likely in tightly packed glia and axons typical of undamaged white matter. We do not know if this modest orientation shift in undamaged white matter has any bearing on the recovery from SCI.

In summary, applied voltages in vivo have been shown to (1) induce CNS nerve regeneration in the mammalian spinal cord, (2) orient the growing fibers, (3) reduce the density of scar forming glial cells crowding into the injury site, but (4) not to influence the density of macrophages also accumulating in the lesion in response to injury.

12 Recovery of the CTM Reflex in Spinal-Injured Guinea Pigs After Exposure to Applied Extracellular Voltages

Implantable stimulator systems similar to those used in anatomical studies were used in tests designed to see if applied voltages could produce behavioral recovery of the CTM reflex. Since the CTM receptive fields are bilaterally organized (refer to Fig. 10), a complete transection of the right side of the spinal cord eliminated the CTM reflex on the right side of the animal below the level of the lesion. This technique was employed in several studies where the intact left side of the spinal cord was associated with a functioning left CTM receptive field. The receptive fields above and ipsilateral to the lesion were also unaffected by the hemisection. This allowed the animal to serve as its own control (Borgens et al. 1987, 1990). Please recall that severing the ascending CTM nerve tract eliminates the reflex for the life of the animal. One hundred percent of untreated control animals do not spontaneously recover this reflex for observation times over 1 year (see Borgens et al. 1993a).

In this series of experiments, active and sham stimulators were implanted subsequent to the transection of the right side of the spinal cord (right lateral hemisection). We had earlier studied several dosages of current (Borgens et al. 1986b), and settled on devices that delivered 35 µA total current for ~ 4 weeks, producing an electrical field around the spinal cord lesion of approximately 300–400 µV/mm (Borgens et al. 1990; Fig. 22).

Current-treated and sham-treated control animals were evaluated for the next 2–3 months using videotaped behavioral analysis and reconstruction of the normal CTM receptive fields and the region of areflexia produced by the injury. We also documented the loss and recovery of the reflex by electromyography. I summarize the results of two separate investigations.

1. A variable level of CTM behavioral recovery occurred in up to roughly 25% of the treated guinea pigs in which the cathode was located rostral to the injury (so as to induce regeneration of ascending CTM spinal cord axons; Borgens et al. 1987, 1990).
2. Sham-treated animals never recovered the CTM reflex. The difference between the two groups was statistically significant (Borgens et al. 1987, 1990).
3. When the anode (or positive electrode) was positioned rostral to the plane of transection, CTM recovery did not occur (Borgens et al. 1990). This was the wrong polarity to influence ascending nerve growth. The correct polarity to influence ascending fibers is to place the cathode out in front of them.

4. When the treatment was delayed for about 3 months following spinal cord hemi-section, CTM recovery did not occur (Borgens et al. 1993a).
5. Behavioral recovery of the CTM reflex was associated with a regeneration of right lateral axons in a region of the ventrolateral spinal cord where CTM spinal cord fiber tracts have been identified (Borgens et al. 1990; Borgens 1992).

These studies provide clear evidence that a functional recovery of a specific behavior, dependent on a known tract of spinal cord axons, could be achieved with an applied voltage gradient of the correct polarity.

A second laboratory confirmed the restorative ability of an extracellular voltage gradient by employing similar implantable stimulators, testing their effect on rat spinal cord compression injuries. Wallace et al. (1987) reported an enhanced performance of rats in response to an imposed DC field subsequent to severe compression injury of their spinal cords. An inclined plane test was used to measure behavioral recovery (Wallace et al. 1987; Fehlings et al. 1988). I have been critical of this type of performance testing (see Chap. 5, "Concerning Behavioral Models for Spinal Cord Injury in Animals"), so "what is good for the goose is good for the gander," and one should not use these behavioral data in support of the hypothesis that applied voltages induce recovery of function from SCI. However, in the latter report, Charles Tator and his colleagues clearly demonstrated the rescue of descending nerve tracts originating from the brain. In untreated control animals, these descending axons were compromised and degenerated following the compression injury. A statistically enhanced sparing of axons was revealed by the enhanced labeling of nerve cells in the brain within the red nucleus, raphe nucleus, medullary reticular formation, and the lateral vestibular nucleus. Neurons in these regions project axons to the level of spinal compression. The technique was foolproof since the HRP marker was applied caudal to the level of the compression injury and labeled a statistically greater number of neurons in the brain than in controls. This result did not discriminate between the possibilities of regeneration, collateral sprouting, or enhanced sealing or sparing of axons in current-treated cords. It did, however, provide solid evidence of a beneficial effect of the applied voltage, sparing important descending projections not previously demonstrated.

13 From a Laboratory Tool to a Clinical Application

All of the studies in rats and guinea pigs noted above, save one, have been conducted using the imposition of DC electrical fields. That is all that is required if one is studying the effects of one polarity of voltage applied across axons of one projection, or a behavior (such as the CTM reflex), dependent on spinal cord axons that are of one projection within white matter. While this has been a good way to explore the biology of applied voltages and nerve regeneration in animals, a clinical tool would not be obvious from such techniques, especially in the injured spinal cord where regeneration of both ascending and descending projections are required within the long tracts.

McCaig (1987) reported that the latency in the response of growth cones facing the cathode was strikingly different than the onset of degenerative changes in growth cones facing the anode of the extracellular voltage. Recall that the responses of nerve processes in vitro are indeed polarized. If neurites grow towards the cathode, they are repelled by the anode. This observation is important to understanding the basis of a clinical technique called oscillating field stimulation (OFS), where the tips of nerve fibers facing in opposite directions may all be induced to extend themselves by regeneration. Cathodally facing nerve processes projecting from single cells in culture begin to show extensions of their growth cone membranes towards this pole within minutes of exposure to the electrical field (Patel and Poo 1982; McCaig 1986). The retraction of the neurites when facing the opposite pole (positive pole or anode) begins on the order of 45 min following field exposure in amphibian neurons at room temperature. This asymmetric response provides a means to direct nerve growth in both directions if the polarity of the field is reversed every 15–30 min (see also Borgens and McCaig 1989). We have tested this proposition in guinea pig spinal cord by combining a miniaturized OFS stimulator (see Moriarty and Borgens 2001) with dorsal hemisection of the mid-thoracic guinea pig spinal cord. We evaluated the axonal responses to ascending and descending projections using injections of different colored fluorescent labels applied rostral and caudal of the hemisection. In sham-treated controls, there was considerable retrograde degeneration of labeled ascending and descending axons approximately 100–300 μm from the transection plane by 60 days after injury. In OFS-treated animals, labeled tracts, both ascending and descending, usually projected to the plane of transection, and in a few cases fibers could be traced around or through the lesion (Borgens and Bohnert, unpublished observations).

14 Naturally Occurring Spinal Injury in the Dog as a Model for Humans

The two most common causes of naturally produced spinal cord injury in canines are fracture/dislocation of the vertebral column (usually resulting from vehicle impact) and explosive intervertebral disc herniations. In the former, spinal injury usually results in complete transection of the dog's spinal cord, a condition that is more severe than observed in human clinical cases (with the exception of wartime injuries) (Toombs et al. 1993; Bunge et al. 1993; Tuszynski 1999).

Explosive intervertebral disc herniation in the dog produces a compression/contusion injury similar to the pathology of human SCI. Many breeds of dogs are susceptible to explosive herniation of disc material directly into the spinal cord. These include chrondystrophic breeds, such as the dachshund, beagle, and corgi, though this trauma can occur in other breeds of dogs as well. In sheer numbers, explosive intervertebral disc herniation results in more clinical cases of canine paraplegia than any other insult.

There are anatomical differences between dog and humans that are interesting to consider when comparing SCI in the two. In humans, the spinal cord ends at L1, thus a common injury at the thoracolumbar junction results in nerve root damage, not spinal cord damage. In dog, the spinal cord ends at L5–L6. Injuries at the same level are true spinal cord accidents in the dog. The ligamentous support of the vertebral column in dogs is different than humans, and intervertebral disc herniations result in discs moving into the spinal canal (in dogs) not away from it (as in humans). In humans, herniated discs press on nerve roots causing pain and discomfort, and sometimes paresis. These are not spinal cord injuries. In the dog, explosive traumatic disc herniation is a true spinal cord accident. Discs dislodge and move inward into the cord compressing it (Fig. 25). Disc material is sometimes removed from the cord, which is compressed to less than 25%–30% of its original diameter, sometimes appearing similar to a burst fracture in the human patient. The dog spinal cord occupies more of the space within the vertebral canal relative to humans, thus it is more seriously damaged by compression. For an interesting review comparing these clinical injuries between dog and man see Horelein (1979). Such naturally occurring injuries in the dog are histopathologically similar to those in the human, causing central hemorrhagic necrosis, secondary injury phenomenon, and an identical axis of behavioral deficits in neurologically complete injuries. The conventional medical management of severe spinal cord injuries in dogs is the same as in humans, including:

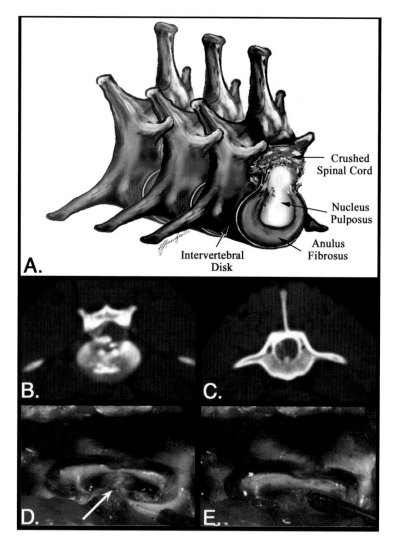

Fig. 25A–E. Disc herniation and spinal cord injury in the dog. The drawing in **A** shows an intervere-bral disc that has ruptured from mechanical force. The soft inner portion of the disc, the nucleus pulposus, is surrounded by a tough fibrous anulus fibrosus that becomes partially mineralized early in the life of some breeds of dogs. Mechanical force can cause disc rupture, extruding portions of the disc into, and crushing, the spinal cord. Most disc ruptures in dog are at the thoracolumbar junction. However, in dog, the spinal cord ends at L5–6, and in humans, L1. Moreover, discs tend to dislodge away from the spinal canal in man, pressing nerve roots, but not in the dog. In **B** and **C**, optical planes in cross-section by CAT reveal the fragmented disc material compressing the cord in the central canal and in a more caudal section at the level of injury in **C**. **C** shows the disc material (faintly) extruded into about 40% of the space formerly occupied by the spinal cord. Intraoperative photographs of a compressed spinal cord are shown in **D** and **E**. In **D**, the disc material (*arrow*) severely compresses the spinal cord. In **E**, note the spinal cord has resumed a more cylindrical shape after this mass has been surgically removed during decompressive surgery, although by this time substantial damage has already occurred in the substance of the spinal cord

110

1. Immediate administration of anti-inflammatory steroids such as methylprednisolone sodium succinate
2. Immediate surgical decompression of the cord by laminectomy procedures (Fig. 25)
3. External stabilization of the vertebral column if required
4. Postsurgical rehabilitation to prevent the fusion of joints and other problems
5. Proper bladder expression and management
6. The use of a wheeled cart to support the hindquarters allowing voluntary locomotion (the equivalent of the wheel chair)

In dogs and in humans, spinal injury may result in lifelong paralysis and interruption in sensory, motor, and autonomic control of bodily functions. For reasons that are unclear, neurologically complete dogs do not usually recover load bearing and ambulation with time after the injury as do laboratory rats, guinea pigs, and cats. If any form of stepping does not appear by about 45–60 days post injury, it never will (see also Henry 1975). Commonly, spinal-injured dogs are euthanized since owners find it difficult to endure the surgical costs and to commit to significant care. However, a small percentage keep their pets for the rest of the animal's lifetime in spite of their injuries. This provides the researcher a pool of both acute and chronically injured dogs with which to test novel treatments. At the Purdue University Veterinary Teaching Hospital (PUVTH) we have followed some paraplegic dogs for 11 years after surgery and their neurological status has not been observed to improve. We have developed a strategy using the naturally injured dogs as a final stage in animal testing before a technique is deemed both safe and beneficial to merit phase I human clinical trials. The inducement to the pet owner to participate is that we pay for all clinical costs, and provide other necessities, such as wheeled carts, as needed.

The afore-mentioned naturally injured chronic dogs were the experimental vehicles permitting rapid movement of 4-AP testing into human clinical trials (see Blight et al. 1991, then Hansebout et al. 1993; Hayes 1994) and more recently the movement of OFS (Borgens et al. 1993, 1999) into human clinical trials at Indiana University Medical Center, Indianapolis, Indiana.

14.1
Clinical Trials of OFS in the Paraplegic Dog

A means to screen incoming referrals of spinal-injured dogs to the PUVTH was developed to include only neurologically complete animals in two separate blinded clinical trials. This process involved rigorous exclusion criteria based on a thorough neurological examination of each candidate and a thorough dialogue with dog owners prior to their signing an informed consent to participate in the study. Neurologically complete paraplegics were defined as being negative on six clinical assessments made prior to surgical decompression of the spinal cord:

1. The complete absence of load bearing and voluntary locomotion in hind limbs.
2. The complete absence of nerve impulse conduction through the spinal cord injury as measured by somatosensory evoked potential testing (a.k.a. SSEP).

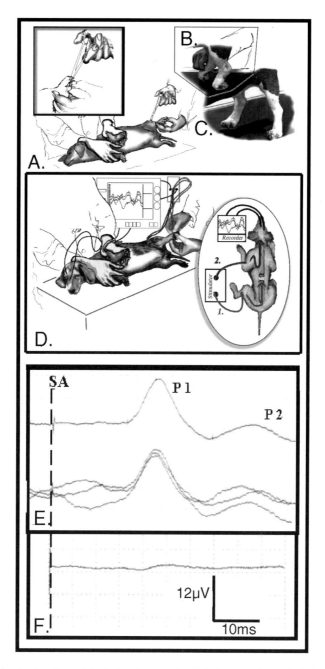

Fig. 26A–F. Behavioral and physiological evaluations in clinical cases of paraplegia in dogs. In **A**, a test for superficial pain is shown, with the neurologist pinching the flank skin below the level of the spinal injury with a hemostat while a helper calms the animal. A positive reaction can be achieved by testing skin above the level of the injury. A third helper videotapes the entire sequence of testing for a permanent record. The *inset* shows a test for deep pain where the joints of the digits are

3. The complete absence of conscious proprioceptive placing of the hind limbs, a test which determines if the animal is aware of the position of its hind paws in space.
4. The complete absence of voluntary micturition (urination) (in the second clinical study monitored by urethral pressure profilometry and bladder cystometry) (Borgens et al. 1999).
5. The complete absence of superficial pain appreciation below the level of the lesion.
6. The complete absence of deep pain appreciation below the level of the injury. (Neurologically, superficial pain can be discriminated by sharp pinching or pricking of the flank skin and hindquarters, while deep pain signals originate from joints, ligaments, and tendons, each are neurologically assessed by different techniques; Fig. 26).

All study animals possessed upper motor neuron signs including normal to hyper-reflexive spinal reflexes. Unlike experimentally induced behavioral loss of the CTM reflex, which never recovers spontaneously, a low frequency of recovery of the various outcome measures is expected in clinical cases of canine SCI. Thus, as in most clinical investigations, blinding and randomization of study animals was important. All of the team members who clinically managed these animals were unaware of the nature of their treatment. Dogs were implanted with active OFS devices or with sham OFS devices. These electronic implants could not be distinguished from each other by even radiography (Borgens et al. 1999). In this second of two studies (Borgens et al. 1999), laboratory fabricated sham and active OFS electronic implants were sent to a corporate sponsor in Warsaw, Indiana for sterilization where they were randomized and coded before being returned to the PUVTH. Thus, no person at Purdue Univer-

◄───

squeezed. Neurologically complete paraplegic animals do not respond to these tests. In **B**, the neurologist turns the rear paw under so that the dorsal surface of the paw rests on the table, while the hindquarters are supported. In a normal dog, the rear paw is immediately returned to a normal stance as shown in **C**. In a paraplegic animal, this test for conscious proprioception is negative and the animals will remain in a knuckled-under stance as in **B**. In **D**, the recording of somatosensory evoked potentials are conducted in a sedated dog. Bipolar stimulating electrodes are inserted into the skin near the tibial nerve of the hind limb (*red*) and/or the medial nerve of the forelimb (*blue*). Electrodes are also inserted into the skin of the scalp, one of the recording electrodes (*black*) over the contralateral sensory cortex relative to the limb stimulated, while the reference electrode can be placed in various places such as the pinna of the ear. The *inset* shows that the stimulation of the median nerve (*blue circuit*) will permit recording of evoked potentials at the brain since the circuit is above the level of the spinal cord injury. Such control-evoked potentials are usually recorded prior to stimulating the tibial nerve. The tibial nerve circuit does not permit evoked potentials to be recorded at the brain since these ascending pathways are interrupted by the spinal cord injury (*inset*). These evoked potential tests are used in both dogs and guinea pigs to test for conduction through the lesion. In **E**, an SSEP record is shown after median nerve stimulation (*SA*, the stimulus artifact). The top trace is an average signal derived from the three individual traces below, evoked by 200 stimulations at 3 Hz (3 mA square wave, 200 μs in duration). *Below* (**F**) is the averaged signal in response to tibial nerve stimulation in the same spinal injured dog shown in E. The injury eliminated the conductance of evoked potentials through the lesion

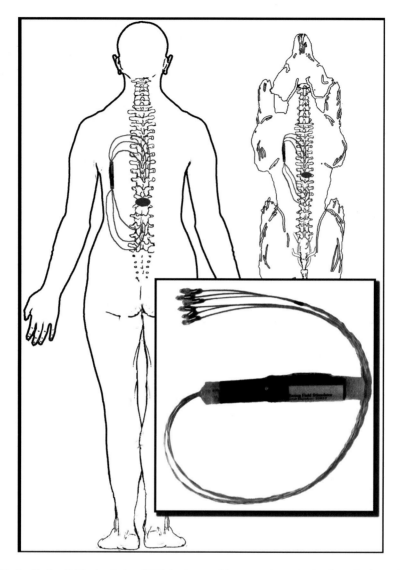

Fig. 27. Oscillating field stimulation (*OFS*) in dogs and humans. An OFS stimulator is shown in the *inset*. These units are currently undergoing FDA-approved phase I tests in severe acute human spinal cord injury at the Indiana University Medical Center, Indianapolis, Indiana. Making sure the dosage of the electrical field was similar in humans to that which proved effective in early trials of canine paraplegia (Borgens et al. 1993) required a design change in OFS stimulators. Since the human's cross-sectional area is about three times that of the small-to-medium-sized dogs used in these early trials, the output of the stimulator had to be increased by about threefold to maintain roughly the same electrical field strength at the lesion. This could not be accomplished by simply increasing the total current threefold since this would produce current densities at the electrodes that would be un-acceptable in soft tissues. Therefore, three independent circuits using three pairs of electrodes were designed (each producing the same level of current as in Borgens et al. 1993), so that the polarity of the field would oscillate at the same duty cycle for all. This new design was tested in dogs and pub-lished in Borgens et al. 1999. The drawing shows the relative placement of the OFS stimulator in the

sity knew the identity of these applications. The code was broken in Warsaw, Indiana only after all neurological assessments were made, and all data tabulated. OFS units were implanted in pockets formed in the musculature just beneath the back skin, and the electrodes routed to a position approximately two vertebral segments rostral, and two vertebral segments caudal to the site of injury, as determined by radiography and by surgical exploration. A unit designed for human use was tested in the second of two clinical trials (Borgens et al. 1999) and is shown in Fig. 27. Behavioral evaluations were made within the first week after surgery prior to the animals being returned to their owners. Animals were returned to the clinic for a complete neurological and radiological evaluation at about 6 weeks and 6–8 months after surgery.

14.2
Recovery of Function in Paraplegic Dogs

The measurements of behavioral outcomes were a part of each neurological examination at 1 week, 6–8 week, and 6-month rechecks. Five measures in the neurological exam were used to determine the extent of functional recovery:

1. Deep pain appreciation
2. Superficial pain appreciation
3. Conscious proprioception
4. Somatosensory evoked potentials
5. Voluntary locomotion

With regard to the latter, we made no attempt to thoroughly document spinal walking or to claim an understanding of the mechanism underlying improved ambulation in these dogs. We simply scored the capability of dogs to ambulate. All the behaviors were scored on a standard form and evaluated again at the end of the study by a panel of investigators unaware of any dog's treatment. Each routine neurological evaluation was composed of five parts:

1. A standard evaluation of spinal reflexes consisting of tibialis, cranialis, patellar, sciatic, crossed extensor, flexor withdrawal, and the cutaneous trunci muscle (CTM) reflex
2. A behavioral evaluation of walking, hind-limb load bearing, superficial pain appreciation, deep pain sensation, and proprioceptive placing
3. Physiological measurement of urethral pressure profilometry and cystometry (performed by a veterinary clinical urologist)

◀——

musculature of the human back and the routing of the electrodes rostral and caudal of the spinal cord injury (*red circle*). The six electrodes are sutured to paravertebral musculature: a set of three electrodes about 2 vertebral segments rostral to the lesion, and the other set of three electrodes, 2 vertebral segments caudal to the lesion. At each location, two of the electrodes are sutured on either side of the vertebral column, the third at its dorsal aspect. The unit and electrodes are removed approximately 14 weeks after implantation

4. Somatosensory evoked potential (SSEP) testing
5. A radiological examination including a myelogram if required

All reflexes and some behavioral tests were performed separately for each side of the dog's body (Fig. 26).

The results of the first trial of OFS included these findings:

1. The OFS-treated group showed greater improvement in every category of behavioral evaluation than the control (sham-treated) group, with no reverse trends at both the 6- to 8-week and 6-month recheck.
2. An average of all individual scores for all categories of blinded behavioral evaluation (The Combined Neurological Score) was used to compare group outcomes. OFS-treated dogs were significantly more improved at the 6-month recheck period compared to sham-treated control dogs.

The results of the second clinical trial using a human use OFS device (Fig. 27; Borgens et al. 1999) were the following:

1. The OFS-treated group showed greater improvement in every category of functional evaluation than the control (sham-treated) group with no reverse trends at both the 8-week and 6- to 8-month recheck.
2. The Combined Neurological Score showed a strong trend towards significance at the 6-week recheck period. At the 6-month recheck period, the Combined Neurological Score of OFS-treated dogs was statistically significantly improved over that of control dogs. Thus, the results of the second trial corroborated the results of the first.

The operation of OFS units in both trials was excellent, as their functioning was determined following the removal of the units in some dogs of the first trial and all dogs of the second trial (Borgens et al. 1993, 1999). Breakage of electrodes was rare in the first trial (1993) and did not occur following modification of the OFS design in the second trial (1999). Few clinical complications were noted in either trial and none of these were associated with the electric current application. Only three dogs died during both trials, two of these due to an unrelated heart ailment and the other was anesthetized due to progressive lower motor neuron dysfunction. This animal turned out to have been implanted with a sham unit so this progressive loss could not have been due to an active stimulator implantation.

14.3
Combined Results of Both Clinical Trials of OFS

It is instructive to combine and compare the neurological data derived from both canine clinical trials of OFS. This provides both an overview of our total experience to date using this form of treatment in acutely injured dogs and provides a larger number of animals with which to compare outcomes (6–8 weeks, $n=33$ OFS-treated dogs, 25 sham-treated dogs; 6 months, $n=31$, and 25, respectively). Of the five categories of assessment, the difference in proportion between recovering and nonrecovering dogs was statistically significantly different in three categories at the 6-month recheck period (superficial pain, ambulation, and the recovery of conduction of the SSEP; $P \leq 0.02$; Fisher's Exact test for proportions). Only 2 sham-treated dogs of 14 recovered appreciation of superficial pain by the 6-month recheck period, while over half of all OFS-treated study animals recovered this sensation in both trials (19 of 31; $P=0.0001$, Fisher's Exact test). In spite of its use as a prognosticator of functional recovery in canine paraplegia (Tarlov 1957; Toombs and Bauer 1993; see discussion in Borgens et al. 1993b), deep pain appreciation turned out to be a less sensitive indicator in these trials, as numerous animals in both groups recovered this sensation by 6 months after surgery (12 of 25 controls; 22 of 31 OFS-treated animals).

After the conclusion of the 1993 trial, it was clear that the next step was to move OFS techniques to human clinical trials; however, the electronic implants used in laboratory rodents and in our initial canine trial were not up to the standards for human application. For at least 2 years we completely redesigned and tested a new generation of OFS devices that included different polymer coatings, electrode components, and sealing techniques to protect the internal electronic components from body fluids. Helium leak-down tests were required, as well as new fail-safe circuitry (which shuts down stimulator functioning if its output strays from nominal), and protection from environmental electromagnetic and radio waves that might interfere with unit functioning. All of this had to be designed and tested, resulting in a new electrical circuit. Some of these innovations were used in the second trial, published in 1999. The United States Food and Drug Administration approved our design and human use protocol in late 2000, as submitted from the clinical team at Indiana University School of Medicine, Division of Neurosurgery, headed by neurosurgeons, Scott Shapiro and Paul Nelson. The first spinal-injured patient was implanted with an OFS device early in 2001. Presently this phase I trial is still being conducted, with eight patients implanted out of a probable end point of 20 patients. I expect we will finish this clinical trial in 2003, as recruitment of only neurologically complete patients meeting a strict exclusion protocol is going slower than anticipated.

15 Sealing the Breach in Cell Membranes with Hydrophilic Polymers

15.1
Introduction

I have discussed the concept of occult damage to neurons and axons – damage that is initially below the level of anatomical detection. This damage may be in response to stretch injury, mild mechanical insult, or the first stages of membrane disintegration precipitated by hypoxia, anoxia, glucose deprivation (i.e., ischemia) or a reperfusion injury. Here, I will focus on the problem posed by a larger breach in the membrane that can be detected with anatomical methods, and one that is not likely to be sealed by natural repair mechanisms of axons. Secondary axotomy is the likely result of the failure of natural sealing mechanisms.

It has long been understood that certain polymers such as ethylene oxide-propylene oxide-ethylene oxide (EPAN) and polyethylene glycol (PEG) have the ability to fuse several cells together into one when their membranes are touching (Davidson et al. 1976; Davidson and Gerald 1976). In fact, the fusion of lymphocytes and mouse myeloma cells with PEG was the essential step in producing immortal lines of antigen-producing cells permitting the widespread development of monoclonal antibodies. This has sometimes led to the use of the term "fusogen" as applied to polymers and surfactants possessing this capability. These usually share a common characteristic of being strongly amphiphilic and hydrophilic (Nakajima and Ikada 1994). This capability was exploited in other ways in the 1970s and 1980s. For example, PEG has been observed to unite several neuron-like cells (PC 12 cells) to aid in electrophysiological measurements and to fuse single axons in the crayfish and earthworm (O'Lague and Huttner 1980; Bittner et al. 1986). PEG is still used to induce vesicle formation and such models frame the basis for investigating the biophysics and mechanisms of endogenous vesicular fusion (Lentz 1994; Lee and Lentz 1997). Until recently, however, the fusogenic ability of PEG has not been exploited to reconnect and repair severe injuries to mammalian nerve processes since in the 1980s all such attempts had failed (Bittner et al. 1986).

To discriminate a small proportion of axons within white matter that might become fused, it required an improvement in the stimulation/recording technology in organ-cultured CNS tissue. The development of the double sucrose gap isolation and recording chamber for mammalian spinal cord by Riyi Shi and Andrew Blight (1996, 1997) allowed us to attempt these kinds of experiments. In this chamber, long strips (~40 mm) of spinal cord white matter can survive to 48 h while the propagation of

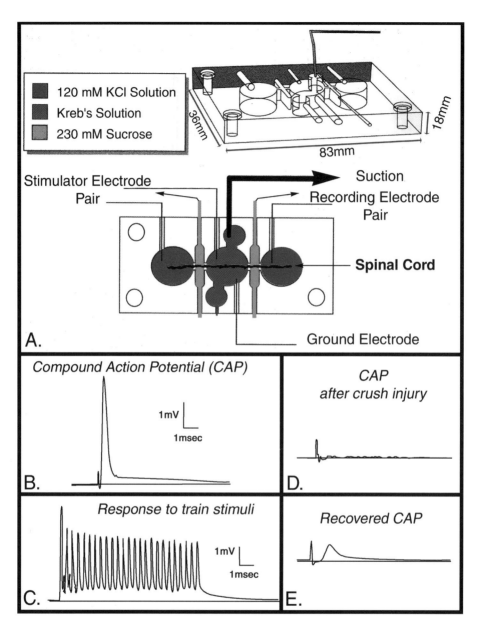

Fig. 28A–E. The double sucrose gap recording chamber. In **A**, the design of the double sucrose gap chamber is shown. The five chambers and their respective media are diagrammed. Sucrose is pumped through the two barrier chambers (*green*) to prevent mixing of the physiological media and to help electrically isolate the ends of the spinal cord, spanning all five chambers. In **B**, a typical compound action potential (*CAP*) is shown, stimulated at one end and recorded at the other. The high resolution of this extracellular recording chamber is represented by multiple trains of CAPs in **C**. In **D**, the elimination of the CAP is shown after a standardized crush of the spinal cord in its middle in the large central chamber filled with physiological Krebs solution (*blue*). A low-magnitude, long-duration recovering CAP is shown in **E**, recorded immediately after a topical application of polyethylene glycol (see text)

compound action potentials (CAPs; stimulated at one end of the chamber and recorded at the other) can be continuously recorded. These measurements are carried out prior to and after a standardized experimental injury to the spinal cord is performed (Fig. 28). Compound membrane potentials (so-called GAP potentials) can also be simultaneously measured in addition to CAPs, providing extraordinary ability to monitor the functioning of injured white matter in the absence of complicating factors such as vascular damage. Strips of spinal cord can be evaluated in this chamber, with gray matter intact or dissected and removed. Double sucrose gap recordings have unequaled signal-to-noise separation allowing even small changes in CAPs to be clearly identified. This was the most important factor in evaluating white matter after damage and during recovery.

15.2
Spinal Cord Fusion: Proof of Concept

Reconnection of proximal and distal segments of spinal cord white matter after complete transection of the cord is not a realistic SCI model. For other reasons though, Riyi Shi and I chose to begin our research into polymer fusion by testing if such a reconnection was even possible. Strips of ventral white matter, approximately 38 mm long, were dissected from adult guinea pigs and placed in the double sucrose gap chamber. Ventral white matter strips (about one-third of the cord's cross-sectional area) were used, as these regions are mainly comprised of large-diameter myelinated axons and possess a more uniform range of axon diameters than the dorsal cord (Shi et al. 1999).

The recording of CAPs traversing the strip were begun immediately after movement of the spinal cord to the sucrose gap chamber and continued constantly through the experiments that usually lasted for a minimum of 2–2.5 h. After the tissue equilibrated in the Krebs medium and CAP recording stabilized, the spinal cord strip was severed into two pieces near its center, roughly 20 mm from either end. This of course completely eliminated the recording of compound nerve impulses stimulated at one end of the strip, and measured when they reached the other end (Fig. 28). The two segments were then reabutted with only slight pressure applied with a laboratory-fabricated utensil maintaining the segments in apposition, but without damaging them further (Shi et al. 1999). An aqueous solution of PEG (~1,800 Da, 50% in water) was applied directly to the transection site with a pipette for approximately 2 min. PEG was then immediately washed off and the region continuously lavaged with Krebs solution as it was pumped through the central compartment of the double sucrose gap chamber. Within 5–10 min, variable magnitudes of CAPs returned. CAPs continued to increase in amplitude with time after treatment. As expected, none of the cords used in control procedures fused or recovered CAP propagation through the transection. The segments of white matter were tightly abutted as in the treatment group, but PEG was not applied in one control group. In the other, cord segments were loosely abutted and PEG was applied as in experimental preparations.

These control procedures checked for a possible alternate pathway for electrical excitation of the distal segment of cord. Furthermore, retransection through the plane of the fusion eliminated *recovered* CAP conduction. As an aside, our initial re-

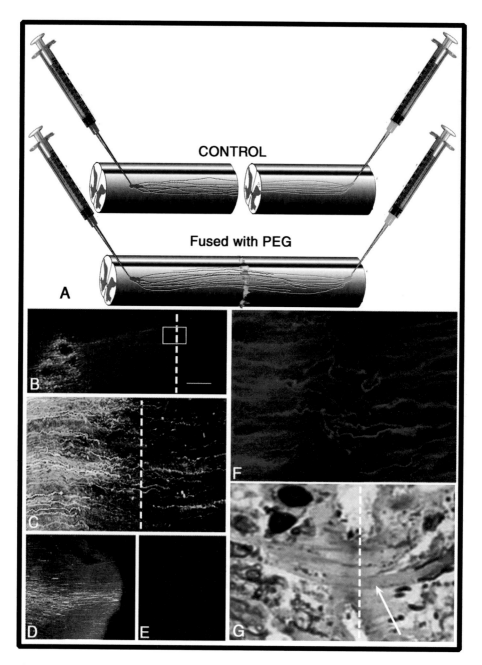

Fig. 29A–G. Axonal fusion in the mammalian spinal cord with polyethylene glycol. In **A**, the drawing shows the two segments of a 40-mm strip of severed spinal cord. In the control cords, the segments were abutted firmly, but PEG was not applied to the transection site. In another set of controls, the segments were loosely abutted, and PEG was applied to the site. In controls and PEG-treated cords, an injection of two fluorescent decorated 8,000 Da dextran markers were made near the end of each segment. On one end, fluoro-ruby was injected, on the other, fluoro-emerald. Though

sults required no practice. PEG application produced immediate fusions and electro-physiological recovery in severed cords.

We next determined if the physiological recovery produced by PEG was associated with anatomical reconnection of axons. Two differently colored fluorescent markers (FITC/dextran and rhodamine/dextran; both 8,000 MW) were injected into the end of each spinal cord segment, one of each color on either side of the transection plane. About 13–18 h was allowed to pass before fixation of the tissues so these markers would be transported within the axons towards the center, where the original tran-section had been performed. In control preparations, axons crossing the transection plane were not observed (Fig. 29D, E). In fact, many axons had pulled back (or de-generated back) into the parenchyma, away from the plane of transection (as in Fig. 11). This occurred as well in some PEG-treated cords; however, variable amounts of axonal reconnection were confirmed since the markers revealed axons spanning the transection plane in both directions. Moreover, numerous axons on one side be-came fused to a single axon on the other, producing anatomies not known to nature (Fig. 29F). Axonal reconnection was also revealed by serial 1-μ-thick plastic imbed-ded sections obtained through the original plane of transection. These showed gross destruction of myelin (and other debris) at the cut, but unmistakable expanses of re-connected axons (Fig. 29G). These experiments proved the capability of PEG to func-tionally and anatomically reconnect the proximal and distal segments of mammalian spinal cord axons.

15.3
Repairing a Crush Injury with PEG

In another series of experiments utilizing the double sucrose gap chamber, spinal cord strips were crushed with a standardized procedure using a motor-controlled impactor. The crush injury to the spinal cord was performed between the stimulating and recording electrodes at its center. The injury was adjusted to be severe enough to eliminate CAP conduction for approximately 45–60 min, but not severe enough to cause secondary axotomy. Natural mechanisms of sealing led to an expected recovery

◀───

the entire spinal cord could be used as drawn, instead, long strips of mainly white matter were used in Shi et al. 1999 to increase the potential to observe fused axons. In B, a low-power fluorescent pho-tomicrograph is shown; the *hatched line* shows the plane of transection and the injection site can be seen (as holes) on the *left*. The *box* marks a region shown in the high-power photomicrograph in C. Note the numerous dye-labeled axons, fused and now continuous across the transection (*hatched line*). In D, a low-power photomicrograph of fluoro-ruby-loaded axons at the plane of transection within the segment injected in a control spinal cord. In E, the corresponding segment of this same unfused control spinal cord showing the complete absence of labeled axons spanning the transec-tion. G is a high-power photomicrograph of a toluidine-blue thin section showing fused portions of myelinated axons (*arrow*) spanning the transection. In F, fluorescent labeling revealed that often sev-eral axons in one segment would fuse to only one axon in the adjacent segment, producing curious whorls of axons such as these. The transection plane is still visible, the hatched line left out so that this anatomy could be easily seen. Images **C–G** are courtesy of the *Journal of Neurotrauma*

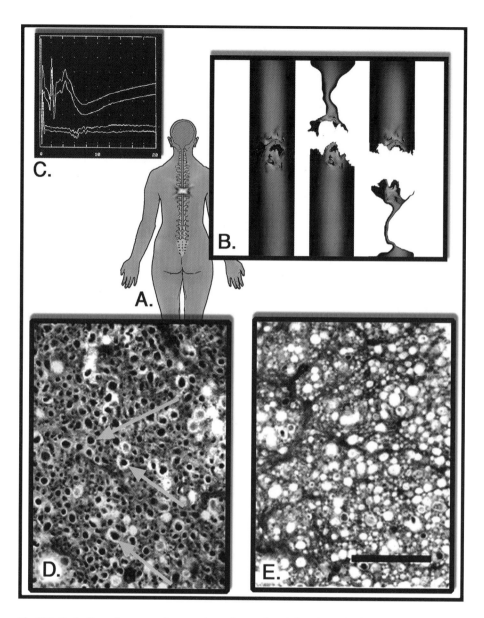

Fig. 30A–E. Sealing of axons and prevention of secondary injury by polyethylene glycol. **A** shows the injury to the spinal cord caused by mechanical compression, typical of the accidents in humans. **B** shows a progression, from *left to right*, of minor breaches in the axonal membrane, which enlarge, causing secondary axotomy in both ascending and descending tracts. The intact portion of the axon remaining after axotomy would be the proximal segment, in continuity with its cell body. This break in conduction interrupts the propagation of nerve impulses through white matter. In **C**, a spinal evoked potential (*SEP*) shows the large magnitude potentials that can be stimulated and recorded within the rostral or caudal segment of cord (*upper pair of traces*), when both pairs of electrodes are located over one or the other segment. **C** shows the substantial reduction in SEPs recorded when the electrodes are placed on either side of the lesion (*lower traces* in **C**). This loss in compound action

124

of a limited amount of physiological function in some control preparations. However, following a 2-min PEG application to the crush site within 15 min of the injury, CAP recovery began 5–15 min after treatment at a time when not one control cord had demonstrated any level of spontaneous recovery. These series of experiments (Shi and Borgens, 1999) proved that membrane breaches sufficient to inhibit impulse conduction could be rapidly restored to function. While the magnitude of the recovered CAPs never reached preinjury values, both their magnitude and latency continued to improve with time.

A dye exclusion test was use to evaluate the hypothesis that PEG anatomically sealed membrane lesions in order to recover conduction. In the first of several experiments, the ability of injured axons to imbibe the intracellular marker horseradish peroxidase (HRP) at the site of local compression of white matter was used as an index of axonal sealing. Axons within the strip of ventral white matter of crushed but untreated spinal cord strips took up the marker and were heavily labeled with HRP. A dramatic reduction in this labeling occurred subsequent to PEG treatment (Shi and Borgens 2000) (Fig. 30). Thus, PEG mechanically repairs damaged nerve membrane sufficient to impede dye uptake while restoring excitability.

Our methods of computer-managed morphometry allowed us to segregate cross sections of individual axons on the basis of their size, from the largest (~5 μm in diameter) to less than 1 μm in diameter. Linear regression analysis of PEG-mediated sealing demonstrated that all sizes of axons were equally susceptible to repair with PEG. HRP is a large molecule (~44,000 Da) which is taken into cells through relatively large holes in the axolemma. We have recently confirmed that PEG seals much smaller breaches, permitting entry of ethidium bromide (~400 Da) into the cytoplasm from the extracellular fluid or the leakage of lactate dehydrogenase (~140,000 Da) out of the cell through the disrupted membrane. PEG seals all such holes (Luo et al. 2002). These experiments also revealed that in control preparations, HRP uptake by injured axons was inversely proportional to the distance from the surface of the cord where contact was made during mechanical compression. This

---

potential propagation through white matter is the biological basis for paraplegia or quadriplegia. Any meaningful recovery of function in humans must be based upon methods that can restore this electrical conduction of nerve impulses through the spinal cord injury. This can occur by providing new circuits through axonal regeneration and/or neurotransplantation – or by preventing the loss of the circuits themselves by interfering or eliminating secondary axotomy – a consequence of progressive secondary injury. In D and E, a means of accomplishing this is shown. In D, a cross section of a severely compressed guinea pig spinal cord white matter is shown. After injury, the lesion was immersed in an HRP label that was taken up into damaged axons through breaches in their membranes. Each individual damaged axon is revealed in this photomicrograph, where the darkly stained axons (*blue arrows*) are surrounded by a light halo of unstained myelin. Note that nearly all of the axons in this cross section were damaged and imbibed dye. In E, a similar injury was treated with PEG within 15 min. Note the striking reduction in axonal injury sufficient to allow uptake of this relatively large marker of approximately 40,000 Da. We have also tested even smaller markers (ethidium bromide) or much larger markers (lactate dehydrogenase, which leaks out of the cell through breaches in the axon). All holes in the axolemma permitting the exchange of intracellular markers are sealed with a brief (2-min) application of the polymer (the scale bar in E, 50 μm). Components of this plate are courtesy of the journal *Neurosurgery* and the *Journal Neurocytology*

very clearly demonstrated the unique character of central damage to the cylinder of spinal cord tissue and its centrifugal spread after compression (Shi and Borgens 2000; shown in Fig. 4).

While physiological functioning was restored by PEG application, axonal membranes had not recovered completely to their preinjury status. CAP amplitudes and other physiological characteristics of conduction remained abnormal for the roughly 1 h of measurement. This included increased refractiveness and a residual and sustained permeability to K^+. The repaired site of damage was still apparently leaky to K^+ since a nearly doubling of the recovered CAP amplitude was produced by subsequent exposure to the K^+ channel blocker, 4-aminopyridine (Shi and Borgens 1999). By the end of 1999, the most important question became whether these striking responses to PEG application could be duplicated in a spinal cord-injured animal.

16 Recovery of Behavioral and Physiological Function In Vivo

Fully adult spinal-injured guinea pigs were the first test subjects for PEG application. We documented the loss and recovery of nerve impulse conduction through the lesion by SSEPs (Fig. 26). The CTM behavior was used to index functional loss and recovery (Fig. 10). These studies began with a topical application of PEG to the exposed spinal cord lesion at various times after spinal cord injury. Electrophysiological and quantitative behavioral records were obtained from each animal prior to a standardized spinal cord compression/contusion injury, immediately after the injury, and at various times after that for 1 month. The constant displacement injury (Blight 1990) was adjusted so that 100% of the control population never recovered SSEP conduction, and spontaneous recovery of the CTM occurred in less than 20% of the population of injured animals. We first applied PEG roughly 15 min after injury. This determined if the striking and rapid changes observed in vitro could be duplicated in vivo. In these studies, an aqueous PEG solution similar to that used in vitro was applied to the exposed spinal cord injury following a hemilaminectomy, durotomy, and lesioning. This was also applied for about 2 min, after which the PEG solution was aspirated and the region thoroughly lavaged with isotonic saline. In additional studies, it was found that direct application of 50% PEG to uninjured spinal cord parenchyma for extended periods exceeding 5 min produced damage to the spinal cord tissues (Fig. 31).

The brief PEG application produced an impressive recovery of SSEP conduction through the lesion in 100% of PEG-treated animals, and variable amounts of CTM reflex recovery in more than 90% of the treated population. These functional recoveries occurred within a few hours to a few days after treatment. None of the control animals recovered evoked potentials and only about 17% recovered CTM functioning; the difference between controls and experimental animals was markedly statistically significant. Thus, the rapid action of PEG in restoring measurable functions after mechanical SCI, originally tested in vitro, was also observed in a well-defined guinea pig spinal cord injury model.

These identical experimental methods were used again; however, the topical PEG application was delayed for approximately 7–8 h after injury (Borgens and Shi 2000; Borgens et al. 2000). There was little detectable difference in response to the delayed application, suggesting the practicality of using PEG in clinical situations. It was also learned that though some very subtle changes in the functioning of recovered CTM receptive fields were identified in the restored reflex (evaluating the vector and speed of CTM contractions and their latency in response to stimulation), overall, the recov-

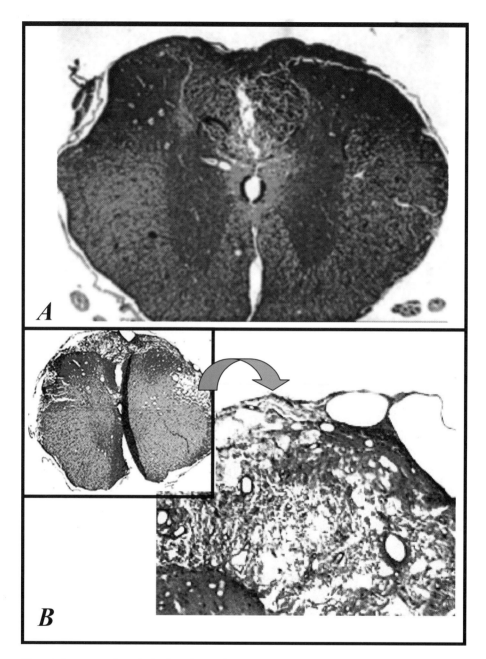

Fig. 31A, B. Destruction of spinal cord tissue by prolonged contact with polyethylene glycol. A brief (<3-min) topical application of PEG (1,800–3,000 Da; 50% by weight in water) can indeed repair holes in axonal membranes and even functionally fuse axon segments together. However, prolonged contact (>5 min) can cause disruption of spinal cord tissue and cavitation. In **A**, a histological cross section of undamaged spinal cord is shown. This section was obtained approximately 1 cm from a topical application of PEG to the same cord (unlesioned and dura removed) for about 5 min. In **B**,

ered CTM behavior was quite characteristic of the original behavior seen prior to injury (Borgens et al. 2002). Actually, one might reasonably suggest that some minor differences in a recovered sensorimotor behavior after its complete elimination by trauma might be expected initially. At least one component of the recovered CTM reflex, its longer latency in response to stimulation, continued to improve with time, approaching the latency typical of the reflex prior to injury.

Three-dimensional reconstruction of the lesion (and adjacent undamaged regions of the spinal cord) was used to evaluate the anatomical responses to immediate and delayed application of PEG. In these visualizations, all serial histological cross sections of the spinal segment containing the lesion were registered and reconstructed using a novel isocontouring algorithm (Duerstock et al. 2000). This allowed not only a realistic 3D view of the tissues, but a quantitative evaluation of many pathological structures imbedded within it. An investigator blinded to the status of the animals carried out both the computer reconstruction and morphometry. PEG treatment produced a statistically significantly reduced amount of gray and white matter damage and reduced the amount of cavitation of the spinal cord. The control lesions were not only more cavitated and cystic, but they were more extended in surface area than the cords treated with PEG. It is reasonable to suggest that an early sealing of the axolemma (or neuron cell membranes for that matter) in a sizable number of cells would reduce the overall inflammatory response, dependent on a progressive accumulation of dying cells. This was our hypothesis, supported by Bradley Duerstock's careful investigation (Duerstock and Borgens 2001). PEG can be considered an antidote to secondary injury. As with any antidote, it appears to work better the sooner it is administered.

16.1
Polymer Injection into the Blood Supply

Using a fluorescently decorated PEG (of approximately 1400 Da), Debra Bohnert and I evaluated PEG's localization in spinal cord crush lesions of adult guinea pigs subsequent to intravenous, intraperitoneal, or subcutaneous injection (Borgens and Bohnert 2001). This was compared to the localization of decorated PEG after topical applications similar to those performed in earlier studies. Undamaged regions of spinal cord were barely labeled, while the lesion was heavily labeled by intravenous or subcutaneous PEG injection. We did not detect a difference in labeling after a 6- to 7-h delayed injection. Apparently, PEG targets the CNS lesion after injury, though the reasons for this specificity are still unclear. An acute injection of PEG might be ex-

---

the *inset* shows a similar cross section at this level and a higher magnification view showing substantial cavitation and destruction of tissue beneath the pia. For this and other reasons of practicality, we no longer use topical applications of PEG, or other polymers such as P188 in spinal cord studies, and instead inject them by intravenous or subcutaneous routes. Administration through the vasculature provides more prolonged contact with damaged tissues at lower concentrations, and better penetration of the polymers into the core of the lesions (see Borgens and Bohnert 2001)

pected to bleed out into regions of CNS hemorrhage. By roughly 7 h after injury, bleeding should have stopped via clotting. Perhaps PEG solubilizes delicate regions of newly repaired capillaries, moving into the extracellular space. At any rate, this was a fortunate observation, as later SCI experiments would use a single subcutaneous injection of PEG 6 h after spinal injury in adult guinea pigs (Borgens and Bohnert 2001). The behavioral and physiological results after a delayed subcutaneous injection of PEG proved to be identical to the acute topical applications. In fact, in this study, the method of injury produced even worse outcomes in control animals. Not one sham-treated control animal recovered any measurable CTM functioning during the 2 months of observation while more than 90% of PEG-treated animals did. The recovery rate after PEG treatment remained at 100% compared to the complete failure of SSEP conduction in controls (compare Borgens and Bohnert 2001 with Borgens et al. 2002 and Borgens and Shi 2000). It should be emphasized that the investigators carrying out behavioral and physiological measurements were blinded to the experimental status of the animals. Even the injections were blinded, the syringe loaded with a PEG or control solution was prepared and coded by one technician prior to passing it on to the surgeon.

16.2
Safety of Intravenous Polyethylene Glycol

The Food and Drug Administration (FDA) considers PEG nontoxic. Its medical uses are numerous and varied including coatings for so-called stealth liposomes, a carrier (solvent) for contrast media, as well as lipophilic compounds such as hemopoietic factors. There is a literature on the IV administration of free PEG in laboratory rodents, rabbits, dogs, and humans dating back some 40 years (for example, see Johnson et al. 1971; reviewed by Working et al. 1997).

PEG is a polymer comprised of ethylene glycol subunits. The monomer is toxic with characteristic clinical signs in both humans and pets (who like to drink automobile antifreeze since ethylene glycol has a sweet taste.) Very-low-molecular-weight PEGs are broken down into individual subunits by a variety of enzyme systems, producing toxicity and symptoms similar to ethylene glycol poisoning (Working et al. 1997). The safety of PEG during parenteral administration is derived from many factors secondary to its long-chain polymeric form. For example, long-chain PEGs (greater than 1,000 Da) are not easily absorbed from the GI tract, and they are cleared at the level of the kidney in the relative absence of participation by renal tubular filtration (generally passed at the level of the glomerulus). Generally, IV PEGs are excreted in the feces and urine in a matter of hours as still large molecular-weight breakdown products. PEG (4,000 Da) has been safely administered in 10% IV solutions to rats, guinea pigs, rabbits, and monkeys at dose levels up to 16 g/kg of body weight. It is also used as gastric lavage in man, passed through the digestive tract in large amounts.

In toxicity studies using dogs, increasing concentrations of PEG (4,000 Da) were administered IV until achieving lethal respiratory arrest. It was noted that the first toxic signs of decreased blood pressure and reduced respiratory rate were both reversible with cessation of administration, and these occurred at a dosage of up to 3 g/kg body weight, causing death at concentrations much greater than this.

Indeed, IV PEG has long been used in humans, and it might be prudent to at least cite the comments of researchers who used PEG as a carrier for antihemophilic factor, infused by IV routinely into hemophilic patients over 30 years ago (Johnson et al. 1971): "during the last two decades, the linear polymers PEG 4000 and PEG 6000 have become purer and are now virtually non-toxic in animals, perhaps because of increasing purity of the ethylene glycol used in the starting material... Toxic effects have not been shown by: repeated intravenous administration over 1 year in beagles, and skin sensitization in animals; renal excretion studies in animals and in man; tests for carcinogenic potential; skin sensitization in man; and equilibrium dialysis experiments for possible protein binding. PEG 4000 is also employed in drugs for parenteral injection (Depo-Medrol, Depo-Provera and NeoCortef – Upjohn Co., Kalamazoo, Mich.,)."

The only reported cases of fatal PEG toxicity in humans that I am aware of, were secondary to its use as a topical creme application to severe burns (see Working et al. 1997). This was deduced to be caused by the continuous application of the low-molecular-weight fraction of the antimicrobial creme (PEG, 300 Da), which produced symptoms similar to ethylene glycol toxicity. In a sentence, the toxicity of PEG is inversely proportional to its molecular weight.

17 PEG Application in Clinical Cases of Canine Paraplegia

Given the positive results gained from studies of guinea pig, veterinary clinical trials of PEG injections as a treatment for severe acute canine paraplegia have just been completed in a joint clinical trial at the Schools of Veterinary Medicine at Purdue University and Texas A&M University. The investigative protocol was similar to that described for OFS studies described in Sect. 14.1. Following admission to the hospital and a standardized neurological examination, to set a baseline of functional and physiological deficits, PEG was administered intravenously as soon as possible to spinal-injured dogs before and after surgery. If a durotomy was necessary, during decompressive surgery PEG was also topically applied to the exposed lesion for 2 min, removed, and lavaged, as in the laboratory experiments discussed in Sect. 15.3 "Repairing a crush Injury with PEG."

The results of this veterinary clinical study will be reported in detail in 2003; however, before providing a summary of our findings, an interesting digression.

We were not able to use concurrent control animals in this trial, and instead had to rely upon historical controls. These control dogs were neurologically complete paraplegic dogs that were part of published trials of the 1990s conducted by the Center for Paralysis Research and The Department of Veterinary Clinical Sciences at Purdue University. We have always used control animals in every canine clinical trial, where an unknown frequency of recovery is expected in response to conventional clinical management (for example, see Borgens et al. 1993, 1999). The use of historical controls in the recently completed PEG trial will likely impact some readers negatively. Nevertheless, the reasons for our collective decision to forego control injections of sterile saline is compelling, I believe, and in my opinion strengthens the case for a rapid movement of polymer infusions into the human clinic.

Before opening the clinical trial for recruitment of severe, neurologically complete canine SCI cases, we sought to develop a protocol for PEG administration in late 2001, and applications were tried on three severely spinal cord-injured dogs admitted to the PUVTH.

Each of these animals recovered substantial motor and sensory function (as well as continence) within 7–10 days of PEG administration. Two animals were standing and stepping before their stitches were removed from incisions after decompression surgery. Two of the three dogs recovered deep and some superficial pain within 10–20 h after surgery. Finally, a large retriever that had sustained the most serious and intractable type of spinal injury seen in the small animal clinic (fracture dislocation of the spine secondary to automobile impact), recovered low-magnitude and long-duration SSEPs while on the examination table during the 15-min slow-push injection of PEG. As a group, we have evaluated over 400 spinal cord-injured dogs during our various studies using this model since 1986, and had never observed such dramatic and rapid changes in function in even incomplete spinal injuries.

The consequence of these pilot administrations of PEG was that the participating neurosurgeons felt it unethical to inject sterile saline (as a control procedure) into neurologically complete paraplegic dogs, knowing full well they will sustain major behavioral deficits for the rest of their lives (Henry 1975). We do not often think such ethical considerations are made in the coarse of experimental animal medicine; however, for the professional veterinary researcher, compassion for both the animal and the clients indeed guide similar sorts of decisions as in human clinical trials.

As a group (36 dogs for comparison, up to 4 days after surgery, and 24 dogs, up to the 6-week recheck), all of these historical control dogs were admitted under an identical clinical protocol; they received the same "standard of care" veterinary management (methylprednisolone sodium succinate injection, decompressive surgery, and spinal stabilization, when required). All controls met an identical exclusion criteria as used to recruit PEG-treated dogs; were admitted about the same time after injury and were of a similar weight and level of injury. Furthermore, the complete medical records and videotapes of all of these previous examinations were available for study. The neurological scores for historical controls were produced by a panel of investigators blinded to the experimental status of any dog, four of whom participated in the current PEG trial. The range of possible scores was 4 (neurologically complete paraplegic) to 20 (a completely normal animal; see Borgens et al. 1999 for details of behavioral and neurological testing). By the end of the 6-week period of study, PEG-treated dogs were strikingly improved relative to controls, documented by a significant difference in the total neurological score and by comparisons between each category of outcome measure. For example, only 4% of all control dogs showed a recovery of proprioception by 6 weeks versus 37% of PEG-treated dogs; 70% of the PEG-treated dogs could ambulate effectively by 6 weeks compared to 25% of controls; 62% of the control population remained neurologically complete paraplegics 6 weeks after surgery compared to only 16% of the experimental group.

At the 6-week recheck, and still later at a 6-month evaluation, three PEG-treated dogs could not be easily distinguished from normal animals except by thorough neurological exam. Only 2 of the 14 control dogs that could be monitored for SSEPs recovered conduction. Seven of the 11 dogs available for testing in the PEG-treated groups recovered ascending conduction, and all 4 of the PEG-treated animals with the highest total neurological scores regained SSEPs (SSEP testing requires sedation, which could not be performed on every dog at every checkup for a variety of reasons). In summary, both the proportions of PEG-treated animals recovering individual behavioral outcome measures, and their mean neurological scores, were markedly statistically significantly improved over controls at all time points (3–4 days after surgery, 1 week and 6–8 weeks after surgery). We chose to end the study at 6–8 weeks without including 6- to 8-month rechecks as in past trials, since the level of improvement in response to PEG was so complete and rapid.

We have also injected another polymer, the triblock surfactant, poloxamer P188, in seven similar cases of SCI in dogs using an identical protocol. All but one animal has responded to this polymer in a manner similar to PEG. Though this observation is of course preliminary, there may be special considerations that may make P188 useful in planned human use.

17.1
The Amphiphilic Triblock Copolymers

There are several interesting experiments in recent years suggesting a more widespread utility of polymer application in various forms of injury. What these injuries have in common is that the initial pathology is due to the instability of the membrane. One of the most interesting is electric shock-induced myonecrosis of muscle.

We have all heard of people that survive touching power lines around their home. Many times the thousands of volts discharged into an extremity may lead to a progressive atrophy, eventually requiring amputation. I have always thought that somehow this had to do with heat transfer to the limb, but this is not the case. Heat damage to soft tissue is very localized. Voltage-mediated electroporation of muscle cell membranes is what leads to progressive myonecrosis (Lee et al. 1992a; Maskarinec et al. 2002). In a series of ingenious experiments, Raphael Lee, Memet Toner, Jurgin Hannig, and their colleagues have explored the use of poloxamers and poloxamines in this and other forms of soft tissue trauma. For example, muscle cells were loaded with an intracellular dye, calcein, which then leaks out of the cell after electrical trauma. Application of poloxamine 1107 or poloxamer 188 reduces or eliminates the electropermeabilization of muscle, stopping or reducing the leakage of the dye (Padanlam et al. 1994; Lee et al. 1992b, c). In a similar type of experiment, fibroblasts in vitro can be protected from lethal levels of heat shock by the application of poloxamer 188 (Merchant et al. 1998). Surfactant treatment can also reduce ischemic damage in a testicular reperfusion injury model in rats (Palmer et al. 1998). Finally, the neuroprotection that poloxamers may provide damaged neurons in vitro has been studied by Marks et al. 2001. P188 provided extraordinary neuroprotection to hippocampal and cerebellar neurons in vitro subsequent to excitotoxic and oxidative injury in culture. Several different toxic conditions were explored, including exposure to NMDA, kainite and a form of hydrogen peroxide, all of which produced significant cell death in neurons. P188 provided significant membrane targeted neuroprotection in all cases when the neurons were incubated in P188 after the toxic test substance.

The triblock polymers are so named because one block represented by PEG chains is linked to a head group (a second block is represented in this case by polypropylene oxide) and yet a third block by PEG. The polypropylene subunit is hydrophobic, while the PEG components remain strongly hydrophilic. It is thought that the triblock polymers more directly target breaches in cell membranes by insertion of the head group into the hydrophobic interior of the membrane exposed by injury (Marks et al. 2001). Thus, some sealing may occur by this hydrophobic interaction, acting in concert with the hydrophilic action of the PEG side chains, which likely reorganize the aqueous phase of the membrane as described in Fig. 32. Interestingly, as the membrane undergoes reorganization to a more normal state, the surface pressure (that all membranes possess) also increases in magnitude to normal levels-displacing the poloxamer head group from the original site of damage (Maskarinec 2002).

While PEG may target the hemorrhagic lesion, P188 may do this as well, and in addition, directly target the lesion in the membrane as well. Marks et al. (2001) suggest a free radical scavenging ability of the poloxamer. PEG is not a free radical scavenger per se, but has the ability to secondarily reduce the production of reactive oxygen metabolites by its membrane sealing properties (Luo et al. 2002).

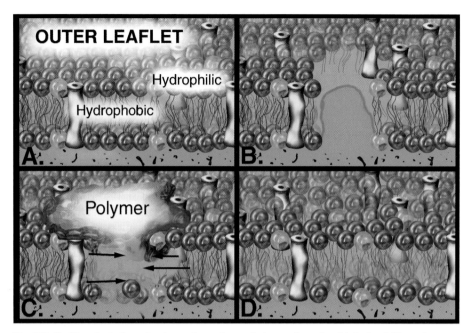

Fig. 32A–D. Hypothetical mechanisms of membrane fusion and repair with hydrophilic surfactants. In **A**, The normal structure of the Danielli–Davson model of the membrane is shown. The hydrophilic outer and inner leaflets sandwich a hydrophobic core of lipidic macromolecules. Various channel proteins and other structures span this membrane. In **B**, a breach in the membrane allows the exchange of fluids and ions across the membrane. In **C**, a strongly hydrophilic surfactant dehydrates the membrane and the interior of the breach. This may allow the hydrophobic elements to flow together, as in the direction of the *arrows*. Other triblock copolymers, such as the poloxamers, insert a hydrophobic core group into the breach (shown in **C**) enhancing both sealing and the formation of a continuous phase in the center of the membrane. The polymers lead to a spontaneous self-assembly of membrane elements as the aqueous phase of the membrane is restored and the increasing surface pressure of the recovering membrane actually dislodges the polymer from its point of insertion (Maskarinec et al. 2002). It is the polar forces associated with the aqueous phase that help support membrane integrity

We have recently completed a long study of P188 injections in the same guinea pig spinal injury model as used in previous PEG investigations (Borgens et al. 2000, 2001). There was no difference in the rate or character of SSEP recovery to a 6-h delayed subcutaneous injection of P188, as was observed in response to a similar injection of PEG in the same injury model (Borgens, Bohnert and Shi, unpublished observations). Recovery of the CTM reflex in response to P188 was significantly enhanced compared to controls, but less impressive than recorded after PEG applications (Borgens and Bohnert, unpublished investigations).

In the clinic, we continue to study this compound, particularly given that it is currently used as a treatment for acute sickle cell anemia in humans, having been administered by IV infusion in massive dosages in over 1000 patients (M. Emanuel, CytRx Corporation, personal communication). Furthermore, the P188 is less viscous than PEG as a working solution, and easier to administer by injection. Plans are currently underway to move one or both of these promising treatments to a phase 1 human pilot study by 2003.

18 Conclusion

Spinal cord injury is a devastating trauma to the body affecting between 10,000 and 12,000 Americans each year. The age of 19 is the most frequently occurring age at injury. Estimates of the chronically injured are harder to deduce; however, it is likely that 250,000–350,000 Americans are severely spinal injured. There are still no effective medical treatments to reverse the considerable behavioral loss that accompanies this type of injury. The standard of care is still decompressive surgery, spinal stabilization, and rehabilitation – treatments that have remained largely the same for over 40 years.

The catastrophic behavioral loss (paraplegia and quadriplegia) results from injury to the white matter of the spinal cord. Only marginal behavioral deficits result from the destruction of gray matter in the majority of clinical injuries in man. The damage to the cord is caused by its compression, rather than transection in most cases, and the region of compromised spinal tissue extends longitudinally less than one vertebral segment. A variable rind of nonfunctional, but anatomically intact, white matter usually remains beneath the pial surface in clinical injuries.

The initial insult to the cord (the primary injury) is followed by a variable but progressive period of continuing dissolution of spinal cord tissue (the secondary injury). Secondary injury is initiated by the disruption of the ionic milieu inside and outside of the cells residing in the zone of injury. Subsequent to ionic derangement, secondary injury is characterized by progressive and self-reinforcing pathological biochemical reactions, hemorrhagic, endocrinological, inflammatory, and other cellular pathologies, which in concert, contribute to the self-destruction of the spinal cord.

Interference with secondary injury mechanisms in the acute phase of spinal cord injury has been an emphasis in clinical research. Reduction of these damaging processes was originally believed to occur in response to intravenous administration of the glucocorticoid methylprednisolone (MP) if administered within 8 h of a spinal cord injury. Early optimism relative to the success of this procedure is fading however, due in part to the modest protection afforded by the required massive dosages of MP balanced against increased side effects and mortality.

Secondary injury can also be reduced through rapid sealing of the membranes of damaged cells by the application of hydrophilic polymers and surfactants. Such intravenous administration of either polyethylene glycol or the nonionic detergent poloxamer 188, cannot only rescue injured nerves and their processes, but as well, rapidly (within minutes) restore physiological function and behavioral recovery in both spinal laboratory animals and clinical cases of paraplegia in canines. This technique is now within months of beginning phase I human clinical trials.

Another means to restore variable levels and types of behavior, lost for extended periods of time after injury in both dogs and humans, is to promote nerve impulse conduction through regions of spared, but nonfunctional, white matter. Said another way, this method seeks to overcome nerve impulse conduction block at the lesion. This can be accomplished by systemic potassium channel blockade through administration of the drug 4-aminopyridine (4-AP), now entering phase III multicenter human trials in North America

In addition to nerve impulse conduction block, the biological basis for the loss of function after spinal cord injury is the break in the nerve impulse conduction pathways by the actual degeneration of the distal segment of injured nerve fibers subsequent to secondary axotomy. Moreover, though regeneration of these amputated processes may begin shortly after injury, in mammals such renewed growth is short lived. This failure of substantive axonal regeneration and synaptogenesis is widely held to be responsible for behavioral loss in the central nervous system of mammals, but curiously, not in their peripheral nervous systems, or in the CNS of many non-mammalian vertebrate animals

There have been numerous claims of facilitated axonal regeneration resulting in behavioral recovery in response to many different experimental treatments in laboratory animals. In the vast majority of these experiments, the data are not at all compelling, corrupted as they are by ambiguous anatomical techniques and inappropriate behavioral analysis. Historically, the use of pyromen and various enzyme treatments meant to reduce scar tissue are typical of early experimental failures. In spite of their popularity, the application of antibodies to block the action of myelin-associated proteins (that are inhibitory to axonal growth and regeneration), the implantation of numerous intercostal peripheral nerve bridges to reconnect the isolated segments of transected spinal cords, and the implantation of neural stem cells are typical of questionable, likely erroneous, claims of beneficial anatomical and/or functional change in laboratory animal models of spinal cord injury in the modern literature.

Modern techniques that clearly demonstrate an ability to both initiate, perhaps guide, nerve fiber regeneration after spinal injury include the application of a steady, weak extracellular voltage gradient and the neurotransplantation of fetal nervous tissue. The supportive anatomical and behavioral bases for these claims, though unambiguous, is scant, relative to the large number of possibly responding neurons and axons surviving near the site of injury. Both of these techniques are now in phase I human clinical trials.

The administration of 4-AP, nonionic detergents and polymers, and the application of exogenous gradients of voltage share a common origin in studies of the biophysics and physiology of spinal cord injury. As experimental treatments, they stand apart from the more conventional approaches born of neurotransplantation and biochemistry. Many conceptions of possible human treatments stemming from the latter may not be clinically practical, and this perhaps provides a rationale for the relatively rapid development of the former approaches, applied as possible clinical therapies for spinal injury in humans.

Coda

It is important to emphasize that the various modern techniques, and ones yet to be discovered, will likely be required to be used in combination(s) to restore significant function and quality of life to the victims of spinal cord injury. It is irresponsible to suggest a complete cure for the conditions of paraplegia or quadriplegia is yet within our reach, in this, or likely the next generation of medical researchers. However, this does not, and should not, detract from the worthy and achievable goal of improving the quality of the injured person's lives, the personal independence that can accompany even modest, yet incomplete, behavioral recovery, freedom from pain, spasticity, the restitution of more voluntary control of bodily functions and vast improvement in the injured person's overall health after this most devastating of human injuries.

References

Albin MS, White RJ, Yashon D, Harris S (1969) Effects of localized cooling on spinal cord trauma. J Trauma 9:1000–1008

Allen AR (1911) Surgery of experimental lesions of spinal cord equivalent to crush injury of fracture dislocation: Preliminary report. JAMA 57:878–880

Allen GH, Ahn HS, Preziosi TJ et al (1983) Cerebral arterial spasm – a controlled trial of nimodipine in patients with subarachnoid hemorrhage. N Eng J Med 308:619–624

Altizer AM, Moriarty LJ, Bell SM, Schreiner CM, Scott WJ, Borgens RB (2001) Endogenous electric current is associated with normal development of the vertebrate limb. Dev Dyn 221:391–401

Anderson MJ, Waxman SG (1983) Regeneration of spinal neurons in inframammalian vertebrates. Morph Develop Asp 24:371–398

Anderson MJ, Waxman SG, Laufer M (1983) Fine structure of regenerated ependyma and spinal cord in stenarchus albiferons. Anat Rec 205:73–83

Arteta JL (1956) Research on the regeneration of the spinal cord in the cat submitted to the action of pyrogenous substances (5 or 3895) of bacterial origin. J Comp Neurol 105:171–184

Auer LM (1984) Acute operation and preventative nimodipine improve outcome in patients with ruptured cerebral aneurysms. Neurosurgery 15:57–66

Barbeau H, Norman K, Fung J, Visintin M, Ladouceur M (1998) Does neurorehabilitation play a role in the recovery of walking in neurological populations? In: Kiehn O (ed) Humans in neuronal mechanisms for generating locomotor activity. Ann NY Acad Sci 860:377–392

Barbeau H, Ladouceur M, Norman K, Pepin A, Leroux A (1999) Walking after spinal cord injury: evaluation, treatment, and functional recovery. Arch Phys Med Rehab 80:225–235

Barde Y-A (1989) Trophic factors and neuronal survival. Neuron 2:1525–1534

Barker AT, Jaffe LF, Vanable JW Jr (1982) The glabrous epidermis of cavies contains a powerful battery. Am J Physiol 242:R358–R366

Barnard JW, Carpenter W(1950) Lack of regeneration in spinal cord of rat. J Neurophysiol 13:222–228

Barnes CD, Worrall N (1968) Re-innervation of spinal cord by cholinergic neurons. J Neurophysiol 31:689–694

Basso DM, Beattie MS, Bresnahan JC (1995) A sensitive and reliable locomotor rating scale for open field testing in rats. J Neurotrauma 12:1–21

Beattie MS, Bresnahan JC, Lopate G (1990) Metamorphosis alters the response to spinal cord transection in Xenopus laevis frogs. J Neurobiol 21:1108–1122

Beattie MS, Bresnahan JC, Komon J, Tovar CA, Van Meter M, Anderson DK, Faden AI, Hsu C-Y, Noble LJ, Salzman S, Young W (1997) Endogenous repair after spinal cord contusion injuries in the rat. Exp Neurol 148:453–463

Bedbrook GM (1987) The development and care of spinal cord paralysis. Paraplegia 25:172–184

Benowitz LI, Goldberg DE, Madsen JR, Soni D, Irwin N (1999) Inosine stimulates extensive axon collateral growth in the rat corticospinal tract after injury. Proc Natl Acad Sci U S A 96:13486–13490

Berkowitz M, O'leary PK, Druse DG, Harvey C (1998) Spinal cord injury: an analysis of medical and societal costs. Demos Med Pub Co NY, NY

Bernstein JJ, Bernstein ME (1967) Effect of glial-ependymal scar and Teflon arrest on the regenerative capacity of goldfish spinal cord. Exp Neurol 19:25–32

Bernstein JJ, Wells MR, Bernstein ME (1978) Spinal cord regeneration: synaptic renewal and neurochemistry. In: Cotman CW (ed) Neuronal plasticity. Raven Press, New York, pp 49–71

Berry M (1979) Regeneration in the central nervous system. In: Smith WT, Cavanaugh JB (eds) Recent advances in neuropathology. Churchill Livingstone, New York, pp 67–111

Berry M, Hall S, Rees L, Carlile J, Wyse JPH (1992) Regeneration in the optic nerve of the adult Browman-Wyse (BW) mutant rat. J Neurocytol 21:426–448

Bixby JL (1999) Molecular mechanisms of axon growth and guidance. Annu Rev Cell Biol 7:117–159

Björklund A (1994) A question of making it work. Nature 367:112–113

Björklund A, Stenevi U (1971) Growth of central catecholamine neurons into smooth muscle grafts in the rat mesencephalon. Brain Res 31:1–20

Björklund A, Stenevi U (1972) Nerve growth factor: stimulation of regenerative growth of central noradrenergic neurons. Science 175:1251–1253

Björklund A, Katzman R, Stenevi U, West KA (1971) Development and growth of axonal sprouts from noradrenaline and 5-Hydroxytryptamine neurons in the rat spinal cord. Brain Res 31:21–33

Björklund A, Nobin A, and Stenevi U (1973) Regeneration of central serotonin neurons after axonal degeneration induced by 5, 6-Dihydroxytryptamine. Brain Res 50:214–220

Blight AR (1985) Delayed demyelination and macrophage invasion: a candidate for secondary cell damage in spinal cord injury. Cen Nerv Sys Tra 2:299–315

Blight AR (1989) Effects of 4-Aminopyridine on axonal conduction block in chronic spinal cord injury. Brain Res Bull 22:47–52

Blight AR (1991a) Morphometric analysis of a model of spinal cord injury in guinea pigs, with behavioral evidence of delayed secondary pathology. J Neurol Sci 103:156–171

Blight AR (1991b) Morphometric analysis of blood vessels in chronic experimental spinal cord injury: hypervascularity and recovery of function. J Neurol Sci 106:158–174

Blight AR (1992) Macrophages and inflammatory damage in spinal cord injury. J Neurotrauma 9:83–91

Blight AR (1993) Remyelination, revascularization, and recovery of function in experimental spinal cord injury. In: Seil FJ (ed) Advances in neurobiology: neural injury and regeneration (vol 59) pp 91–103

Blight AR (1994) Effects of silica on the outcome from experimental spinal cord injury: implication of macrophages in secondary tissue damage. Neuroscience 60:263–273

Blight AR, Decrescito V (1986) Morphometric analysis of experimental spinal cord injury in the cat: the relation of injury intensity to survival of myelinated axons. Neuroscience 19:321–341

Blight AR, Gruner JA (1983) Augmentation by 4-Aminopyridine of vestibulospinal free fall responses in chronic spinal-injured cats. J Neurolog Sci 82:145–159

Blight AR, McGinnis ME, Borgens RB (1990) Cutaneus trunci muscle reflex of the guinea pig. J Comp Neurol 296:614–633

Blight AR, Toombs JP, Bauer MS, Widmer WR (1991) The effects of 4-Aminopyridine on neurological deficits in chronic cases of traumatic spinal cord injury in dogs: a phase I clinical trial. J Neurotrauma 8:103–119

Borgens RB (1977) Skin batteries and limb regeneration. Nat Hist Oct: 85–89

Borgens RB (1982) What is the role of naturally produced electric current in vertebrate regeneration and healing? Int Rev Cytol 76:245–298

Borgens RB (1983) The role of ionic current in the regeneration and development of the amphibian limb. In: Fallon JF, Caplan AI (eds) Proceedings of the 3rd international conference on limb development and regeneration. Alan R Liss, New York, pp 597–608

Borgens RB (1984) Are limb development and limb regeneration both initiated by an integumentary wounding? Differentiation 28:87–93

Borgens RB (1988) Stimulation of neuronal regeneration and development by steady electrical fields. In: Waxman SG (ed) Advances in neurology Vol 47: functional recovery in neurological diseases. Raven Press, New York pp 547–564

Borgens RB (1989) Natural and applied currents in limb regeneration and development. In: Borgens RB, Robinson DR, Vanable JW Jr, McGinnis ME (eds) Electric fields in vertebrate repair. Alan R Liss, New York, pp 27–75

Borgens RB (1989) Artificially controlling axonal regeneration and development by applied electric fields. In: Borgens RB, Robinson KR, Vanable JW Jr, McGinnis ME (eds) Electric fields in vertebrate repair. Alan R Liss New York, pp 117–170

Borgens RB (1992) Applied voltages in spinal cord reconstruction: History, strategies, and behavioral models. In: Illis LS (ed) Spinal cord dysfunction, Vol III: functional stimulation. Oxford Medical Publications, Oxford pp 110–145

Borgens RB (1999) Electrically mediated regeneration and guidance of adult mammalian spinal axons into polymeric channels. Neuroscience 91:251–264

Borgens RB (2001) Cellular engineering: molecular repair of membranes to rescue cells of the damaged nervous system. Neurosurgery 49:370–379

Borgens RB, Bohnert DM (1987) The responses of mammalian spinal axons to an applied DC voltage gradient. Exp Neurol 145:376–389

Borgens RB, Bohnert DM (2001) Rapid recovery from spinal cord injury after subcutaneously administered polyethylene glycol. J Neurosci Res 66:1179–1186

Borgens RB, McCaig CD (1989) Endogenous currents in nerve repair, regeneration, and development. In: Borgens RB, Robinson DR, Vanable JW Jr, McGinnis ME (eds) Electric fields in vertebrate repair. Alan R Liss, Inc. New York pp 77–116

Borgens RB, Shi R (1995) Uncoupling histogenesis from morphogenesis in the vertebrate embryo by collapse of the transneural tube potential. Dev Biol 203:456–467

Borgens RB, Shi R (2000) Immediate recovery from spinal cord injury through molecular repair of nerve membranes with polyethylene glycol. FASEB 14:27–35

Borgens RB, Vanable JW Jr, Jaffe LF (1979) Small artificial currents enhance Xenopus limb regeneration. J Exp Zool 207:217–226

Borgens RB, Vanable JW Jr, Jaffe LF (1979) Reduction of sodium dependent stump currents disturbs Urodele limb regeneration. J Exp Zool 209:377–386

Borgens RB, Jaffe LF, Cohen MJ (1980) Large and persistent electrical currents enter the transected spinal cord of the lamprey eel. Proc Natl Acad Sci U S A 77:1209–1213

Borgens RB, Roederer E, Cohen MJ (1981) Enhanced spinal cord regeneration in lamprey by applied electric fields. Science 213:611–617

Borgens RB, Rouleau MF, DeLanney LE (1983) A steady efflux of ionic current predicts hind limb development in the axolotl. J Exp Zool 228:491–503

Borgens RB, Blight AR, Murphy DJ (1986a) Axonal regeneration in spinal cord injury: a perspective and new technique. J Comp Neurol 250:157–167

Borgens RB, Blight AR, Murphy DJ (1986b) Transected dorsal column axons within the guinea pig spinal cord regenerate in the presence of an applied electric field. J Comp Neurol 250:168–180

Borgens RB, Blight AR, McGinnis ME (1987a) Behavioral recovery induced by applied electric fields after spinal cord hemisection in guinea pig. Science 238:366–369

Borgens RB, Callahan L, Rouleau M (1987b) Anatomy of axolotl flank integument during limb bud development with special reference to a transcutaneous current predicting limb formation. J Exp Zool 244:203–214

Borgens RB, Blight AR, McGinnis ME (1990) Functional recovery after spinal cord hemisection in guinea pigs: the effects of applied electric fields. J Comp Neurol 296:634–653

Borgens RB, Metcalf ME, Blight AR (1993a) Delayed application of direct current electric fields in experimental spinal cord injuries. Restor Neurol Neurosci 5:173–179

Borgens RB, Toombs JP, Blight AR, McGinnis ME, Bauer MS, Widmer WR, Cook JR Jr (1993b) Effects of applied electric fields on clinical cases of complete paraplegia in dogs. Restor Neurol Neurosci 5:305–322

Borgens RB, Shi R, Mohr TJ, Jeager CB (1994) Mammalian cortical astrocytes align themselves in a physiological voltage gradient. Exp Neurol 128:41–49

Borgens RB, Toombs JP, Breur G, Widmer WR, Water D, Harbath AM, March P, Adams LG (1999) An imposed oscillating electrical field improves the recovery of function in neurologically complete paraplegic dogs. J Neurotrauma 16:639–657

Borgens RB, Shi R, Bohnert D (2002) Behavioral recovery from spinal cord injury following delayed application of polyethylene glycol. J Exp Biol 205:1–12

Bracken MB (1992) Pharmacological treatment of acute spinal cord injury: current status and future prospects. Paraplegia 30:102–107

Bracken MB, Holford TR (1993) Effects of timing of methylprednisolone or naloxone administration on recovery of segments and long-tract neurological function in NASCIS 2. J Neurosurg 79:500–507

Bracken MB, Collins WF, Freeman DF, Shepard MJ, Wagner FW, Silten RM, Hellengrand KG, Ransohoff J, Hunt WE, Perot PL, Grossman RG, Green B, Eisenberg HM, Rifkinson N, Goodman JH, Meagher JM, Fischer B, Clifton GL, Flamm ES, Rave SE (1984) Efficacy of methylprednisolone in acute spinal cord injury. JAMA 251:45–52

Bracken MB, Shepard MJ, Hellenbrand K (1985) Methylprednisolone and neurological function one year after spinal cord injury. J Neurosurg 63:704–713

Bracken MB, Shepard MJ, Collins WF, Holford TR, Young W, Baskin DS, Eisenberg HM, Flam E, Leo-Summers L, Maroon J, Marshal LF, Perot PI Jr, Piepmeier J, Sonntag VKH, Wagner FC, Wilberger JE, Winn HR (1990) A randomized, controlled trial of methylprednisolone or naloxone in the treatment of acute spinal-cord injury. N Engl J Med 322:1405–1411

Bracken MB, Shepard MJ, Collins WF Jr, Holford TR, Baskin DS, Eisenberg HM, Flamm E, Leo-Summers L, Maroon JC, Marshall LF (1992) Methylprednisolone or naloxone treatment after acute spinal cord injury: 1 year follow-up data. Results of the second national acute spinal cord injury study. J Neurosurg 76:23–31

Bracken MB, Shepard MJ, Holford TR, Leo-Summers L, Aldrich EF, Fazl M, Fehlings M, Herr DL, Hitchon PW, Marshall LF, Nockels RP, Pascale V, Perot PL Jr, Piepmeier J, Sonntag VK, Wagner F, Wilberger JE, Winn HR, Young W (1997) Administration of methylprednisolone for 24 or 48 hours or tirilazad mesylate for 48 hours in the treatment of acute spinal cord injury. Results of the third national acute spinal cord injury randomized controlled trial. Acute spinal cord injury study. JAMA 277:1597–1604

Bracken MB, Shepard MJ, Holford TR, Leo-Summers L, Aldrich EF, Fazl M, Fehlings MG, Herr DL, Hitchon PW, Marshall LF, Nockels RP, Pascale V, Perot PL Jr, Piempmeier J, Sonntag VKH, Wagner F, Wilberger JE, Winn HR, Young W (1998) Methylprednisolone or tirilazad mesylate administration after acute spinal cord injury: 1-year follow up. Results of the third national acute spinal cord injury randomized controlled trial. J Neurosurg 89:699–706

Bray D (1987) Growth cones: Do they pull or are they pulled? Trends Neurosci 10:431–434

Bray GM, Villegas-Pérez MP, Vidal-Sanz M, Aguayo AJ (1987) The use of peripheral nerve grafts to enhance neuronal survival, promote growth and permit terminal reconnections in the central nervous system of adult rats. J Exp Biol 132:5–19

Britland S, McCaig CD (1996) The response of cultured Xenopus neurites to simultaneous electrical and adhesive guidance cues. Exp Cell Res 226:31–38

Bunge RP, Puckett WR, Becerra JL, Marcillo A, Quencer RM (1993) Observations on the pathology of human spinal cord injury: a review and classification of 22 new cases with details from a case of chronic cord compression with extensive focal demyelination. Adv Neurol 59:75–89

Cai D, Shen Y, DeBellard ME, Tang S, Filbin MT (1999) Prior exposure to neurotrophins blocks inhibition of axonal regeneration by MAG and myelin via a cAMP-dependent mechanism. Neuron 22:89–101

Campbell JC, Bassett CAL, Thurlin CA, Feringa ER (1960) The use of nerve grafts to orient axonal regeneration in transected spinal cords. Anat Rec 136:174

Carafoli E, Crompton M (1976) Calcium ions and mitochondria. In: Duncan CY (ed) Symposium of the society for experimental biology: Calcium and biological systems. (vol 30) Cambridge University Press, New York and London 30 pp 89–115

Caroni P, Schwab ME (1988a) Two membrane protein fractions from rat central myelin with inhibitory properties for neurite growth and fibroblast spreading. J Cell Biol 106:1281–1288

Caroni P, Schwab M (1988b) Antibody against myelin-associated inhibitor of neurite growth, neutralizes nonpermissive substrate properties of CNS white matter. Neuron 1:85–96

Cheng H, Cao Y, Olson L (1996) Spinal cord repair in adult paraplegic rats: partial restoration of hind limb function. Science 273:510–513

Cheng H, Almstrom S, Gimenez-Llort L, Chang R, Orgren SO, Hoffer B, Olson L (1997) Gait analysis of adult paraplegic rats after spinal cord injury. Exp Neurol 148:544–557

Chernoff EAG, Stocum DL (1995) Developmental aspects of spinal cord and limb regeneration. Dev Growth Differ 37:133–147

Chi NH, Bignami A, Bich NT, Dahl D (1980) Autologous sciatic nerve grafts to the rat spinal cord. Immunoflourescent studies with neurofilament and gliofilament (GFA) antiserum. Exp Neurol 68:568–580

Clement CD (1964) Regeneration in the vertebrate central nervous system. Int Rev Neurobiol 6:257–301

Clemente CD (1955) Structural regeneration in the mammalian central nervous system and the role of neuroglia and connective tissue. In: Windle WF (ed) Regeneration in the central nervous system. pp 147–161

Cohan CS, Connor JA, and Kater SB (1987) Electrically and chemically mediated increases in intracellular calcium in neuronal growth cones. J Neurosci 7:3588–3599

Cohen S (1960) Purification of a nerve-growth promoting protein from the mouse salivary gland and its neurocytotoxic antiserum. Proc Natl Acad Sci U S A 46:302–311

Cooper MS, Miller MP, Fraser SE (1989) Electrophoretic repatterning of charged cytoplasmic molecules within tissues by direct current electric fields. J Cell Biol 102:1384–1399

Cotman CW, Cummings BJ, Pike CJ (1992) Molecular cascades in adaptive versus pathological plasticity. In: Gorio A (ed) Neuroregeneration. Raven Press New York, pp 217–240

Cowan SL (1934) The action of potassium and other ions on the injury potential and action current in maia nerve. Proc Royal Soc (London) 3115:216–260

Cowan WM, Fawcett, O'Leary D, Stanfield B (1984) Regressive events in neurogenesis. Science 225:1258–1287

Damoiseaux JG, Dopp EA, Calame W, Choa D, MacPherson GG, Dijkstra CD (1994) Rat macrophage lysosomal membrane antigen recognized by monoclonal antibody ED1. Immunology 83:140–147

Davenport RW, McCaig CD (1993) Hippocampal growth cone responses to focally applied electric fields. J Neurobiol 24:89–100

David S, Aguayo AJ (1981) Axonal elongation into peripheral nervous system "bridges" after central nervous system injury in adult rats. Science 214:931–933

David S, Aguayo AJ (1985) Axonal regeneration after crush injury of rat central nervous system fibres innervating peripheral nerve grafts. J Neurocytol 14:1–12

Davidson RL, Gerald PS (1976) Improved techniques for the induction of mammalian cell hybridization by polyethylene glycol. Somatic Cell Mol Genet 2:165–176

Davidson RL, O'Malley KA, Wheeler TB (1976) Induction of mammalian somatic cell hybridization by polyethylene glycol. Somatic Cell Mol Genet 2:271–280

Davies SJ, Goucher D, Coller C, Silver J (1999) Robust regeneration of adult sensory axons in degenerating white matter of the adult rat spinal cord. J Neurosci 19:5810–5822

Davies SJA, Fitch MT, Memberg SP, Hall AK, Raisman G, Silver J (1997) Regeneration of adult axons in white matter tracts of the central nervous system. Nature 390:680–683

DeVivo MJ, Whiteneck GC, Charles ED Jr (1995) The economic impact of spinal cord injury. In: Stover SL, Delisa JA, Whiteneck GG (eds) Spinal cord injury: clinical outcomes from the model systems. Aspen Publications, Aspen CO, pp 234–271

Dimeitrijevic MR, Gerasimenko Y, Pinter M (1998) Evidence for a spinal central pattern generator in humans. In: Kiehn O (ed) Neuronal mechanisms for generating locomotor activity. Ann N Y Acad Sci 860:360–376

Ditunno JF, Formal CS (1994) Chronic spinal cord injury. N Eng J Med 330:550–556

Donaldson J, Shi R, Borgens R (2002) Polyethylene glycol rapidly restores physiological functions in damaged sciatic nerves of guinea pigs. Neurosurgery 50:147–157

DuBois-Reymond E (1843) Vorlaufiger abrifs einer untersuchung uber den sogenannten froschstrom und uber elie electromotorischen fische. Ann Phys U Chem 58:1–48

Duerstock BS, Borgens RB (2002) Three-dimensional morphometry of spinal cord injury following polyethylene glycol treatment. J Exp Biol 205:13–24

Duerstock BS, Bajaj CL, Pascucci V, Schikore D, Lin K-N, Borgens RB (2000) Advances in three-dimensional reconstructions of the experimental spinal cord injury. Comput Graphics 24:389–406

Duffy MT, Liebich DR, Garner LK, Hawrych A, Simpson SB Jr, Davis BM (1992) Axonal sprouting and frank regeneration in the lizard tail spinal cord: correlation between changes in synaptic circuitry and axonal growth. J Comp Neurol 316:363–374

Eidelberg EJ, Sullivan J, Bingham WC (1975) Immediate consequences of spinal cord injury: possible role of potassium in axonal conduction block. Surg Neurol 3:317–321

Eidelberg EJ, Walden LH, Nguyen LH (1981) Locomotor control in macaque monkeys. Brain 104:647–663

Erskine L, McCaig CD (1995) Growth cone neurotransmitter receptor activation modulates electric field-guided nerve growth. Dev Biol 171:330–339

Erskine L, McCaig CD (1997) Integrated interactions between chondroitin sulphate proteoglycans and weak DC electric fields regulate nerve growth cone guidance in vitro. J Cell Science 110:1957–1965

Faden Al, Jacobs TP, Smith MT (1984) Thyrotropin-releasing hormone in experimental spinal injury: dose response and late treatment. Neurology 34:1280–1284

Faden AI, Salzman S (1992) Pharmacological strategies in CNS trauma. Trends Pharmacol Sci 13:29–35

Faden AI, Yum SW, Lemke M, Vink R (1990) Effects of TRH-analog treatment on tissue cations phospholipids and energy metabolism after spinal cord injury. J Pharmacol Exp Ther 255:608–614

Fawcett JW, Asher RA (1999) The glial scar and central nervous system repair. Brain Res Bull 49:377–391

Fawcett JW, Fersht N, Housden L, Schachner M, Pesheva P (1992) Axonal growth on astrocytes is not inhibited by oligodendrocytes. J Cell Sci 103:571–579

Fawcett JW, Keynes RJ (1990) Peripheral nerve regeneration. Annu Rev Neurosci 13:43–60

Fehlings MG, Tator CH, Linden RD (1988) The effect of direct-current field on recovery from experimental spinal cord injury. J Neurosurg 68:781–792

Feigin E, Geller EH, Wolf A (1951) Absence of regeneration in the spinal cord of the young rat. J Neuropathol Exp Neurol 10:420–425

Fertig A, Kiernan JA, Seyan SS (1971) Enhancement of axonal regeneration in the brain of the rat by corticotrophin and triiodothyronine. Exp Neurol 33:372–385

Fitch M, Silver J (1997) Activated macrophages and the blood-brain barrier: inflammation after CNS injury leads to increases in putative inhibitory molecules. Exp Neurol 148:587–603

Folis F, Scremin OU, Blisard KS, Scremin AM, Pet SB, Scott WJ, Kessler RM, Wernly JA (1993) Selective vulnerability of white matter during spinal cord ischemia. J Cereb Blood Flow Metab 13:170–178

Foerster AP (1982) Spontaneous regeneration of cut axons in adult rat brain. J Comp Neurol 210:335–356

Freed WJ, de Medinaceli, Wyatt RJ (1985) Promoting functional plasticity in the damaged nervous system. Science 227:1544–1552

Freeman LW, Mac Dougall J, Turbes CC, Bowmann DE (1960) The treatment of experimental lesions of the spinal cord of dogs with trypsin. J Neurosurg 17:259–265

Friedman RM, Ritz LA, Reier PJ, Vierck CJ Jr (2000) Effects of sacrocaudal spinal cord transection and transplantation of fetal spinal tissue on withdrawal reflexes of the tail. Neurorehab Neural Repair 14:331–343

Frisen J, Fried K, Sjogren AM, Risling M (1993) Growth of ascending spinal axons in CNS scar tissue. Int J Dev Neurosci 4:461–475

Galabov G (1966) Regeneration of sectioned spinal cord by implantation of a peripheral nerve [in Russian]. Dokl Bolg Akad Nauk 19:449–452

Gelmers HJ (1984) The effects of nimodipine on the clinical course of patients with acute ischemic stroke. Acta Neurol Scand 69:232–239

Geisert E, Yang L, Irwin MH (1996) Astrocyte growth, reactivity, and the target of the antiproliferative antibody, tAPA. J Neurosci 16:5478–5487

146

Geisler FH, Dorsey FC, Coleman WP (1991) Recovery of motor function after spinal cord injury: a randomized placebo-controlled trial with GM-1 ganglioside. N Engl J Med 324:1829–1838

George R, Griffin JW (1994) Delayed macrophage response and myelin clearance during Wallerian degeneration in the central nervous system: the dorsal radiculotomy model. J Exp Neurol 129:225–236

Giovanini MA, Reier PJ, Eskin TA, Wirth E, Anderson DK (1997) Characteristics of human fetal spinal cord grafts in the adult rat spinal cord: influences of lesion and grafting conditions. Exp Neurol 148:523–543

Giugni TD, Braslau DL, Haigler HT (1987) Electric field induced redistribution and post field relaxation of epidermal growth factor receptors on A431 cells. J Cell Biol 104:1291–1297

Giulian R, Chen J, Ingman J, George JK, Noponen M (1989) The role of mononuclear phagocytes in wound healing after traumatic injury to adult mammalian brain. J Neurosci 9:4416–4429

Go BE, DeVivo M, Richards JS (1995) The epidemiology of spinal cord injury. In: Spinal cord injury: clinical outcomes from the model systems. Stover SL, Delisa JA, Whiteneck GG (eds) Aspen Publications, Aspen CO, pp 21–55

Goldberger ME (1980) Motor recovery after lesions. Trends in Neurosci 3:288–298

Goldberger ME, Murray M (1978) Recovery of movement and axonal sprouting may obey some of the same laws. In: Cotman CW (ed) Neuronal plasticity. Raven Press, New York, pp 73–96

Goldberger MM, Murray M, Tessler A (1992) Sprouting and regeneration in the spinal cord: their roles in recovery of function after spinal injury. In: Gorio A (ed) Neuroregeneration. Raven Press, New York, pp 241–265

Goslin K, Banker G (1989) Experimental observations on the development of polarity by hippocampal neurons in culture. J Cell Biol 108:1507–1516

Greitz D, Ericson K, Flodmard O (1999) Pathogenesis and mechanics of spinal cord cysts. Int J Neuroradiol 5:61–78

Grill RJ, Blesch A, Tuszynski MH (1997) Robust growth of chronically injured spinal cord axons induced by grafts of genetically modified NGF-secreting cells. Exp Neurol 148:444–452

Grillner S, Zangger P (1979) On the central generation of locomotion in the low spinal cat. Exp Brain Res 34:241–261

Grillner S, Ekeberg O, El Manira A, Lansner A, Parker D, Tegner J, Wallen P (1998) Intrinsic function of a neuronal network: a vertebrate central pattern generator. Brain Res Rev 26:184–197

Gundersen RW, Barrett JN (1980) Characterization of the turning response of dorsal root neurites toward nerve growth factor. J Cell Biol 87:546–554

Guth L, Bright D, Donati EJ (1978) Functional deficits and anatomical alterations after higher cervical spinal hemisection in the rat. Exp Neurol 58:511–520

Hagins WA (1972) The visual process: excitatory mechanisms in the primary receptor cells. Ann Rev Biophys Bioeng 1:131–158

Hall ED (1992) The neuroprotective pharmacology of methylprednisolone. J Neurosurg 76:13–22

Halter JA, Blight AR, Donovan WH, Calvillo O (2000) Intrathecal administration of 4-Aminopyridine in chronic spinal injured patients. Spinal Cord 12:7828–732

Hansebout RR, Blight AR, Fawcett S, Reddy K (1993) 4-Aminopyridine in chronic spinal cord injury: a controlled, double-blind, crossover study in eight patients. J Neurotrauma 10:19–24

Hatten, ME (1990) Riding the glial monorail: a common mechanism for glial guided neuronal migration in different regions of then developing mammalian brain. Trends Neurosci 13:179–181

Hatten ME, Liem RKH, Shelanski ML, Mason CA (1991) Astroglia in CNS injury. Glia 4:233–243

Hayes KC (1994) 4-Aminopyridine and spinal cord injury: a review. Restor Neurol Neurosci 6:259–270

Hayes KC, Blight AR, Potter PJ, Allat RD, Hsich JTC, Wolfe DL, Lam S, Hamilton JT (1993) Preclinical trial of 4-aminopyridine in patients with chronic spinal cord injury. Paraplegia 31:216–224

Heinicke EA (1980) Vascular permeability and axonal regeneration in tissues autotransplanted into the brain. Acta Neuropathol 49:177–185

Heinicke EA, Kiernan JA (1978) Vascular permeability and axonal regeneration in skin autotransplanted into the brain. J Anat 125:409–420

Herlitzka A (1910) Ein Beitrag zur physiologie der gerneration. Wilhelm Roux Arch 10:126–158

Hinkle L, McCaig CD, Robinson KR (1981) The direction of growth of differentiating neurones and myeloblasts from frog embryos in an applied electric field. J Physiol 314:121–135

Holtz A, Nystrom B, Gerdin B (1989) Spinal cord injury in rats: Inability of nimodipine or anti-neutrophil serum to improve spinal cord blood flow or neurologic status. Acta Neurol Scand 79:460–467

Honmou O, Young W (1995) Traumatic injury of spinal axons. In: Waxman SG, Kocsis JD, Stys PK (eds) The Axon. Oxford University Press, New York, pp 480–529

Horvat JC (1966) Comparison des réactions régénératives provoquées dans le cerveau et dans le cervelet de la souris par des greffes tissulaires intravaciales. C R Assoc Anat (Paris) 51:487–499

Houle JD, Reier P (1988) Transplantation of fetal spinal cord tissue into the chronically injured adult rat spinal cord. J Comp Neurol 269:535–547

Houle JD, Reier P (1989) Regrowth of calcitonin gene-related peptide (CGRP) immonoreactive axons from the chronically injured rat spinal cord into fetal spinal cord tissue transplants. Neurosci Lett 103:253–258

Horvat (1980) Influence des cellules de Schwann greffées sur la régénération des fibres nerveuses intraspinales lors de la transplantation de fragments de nerf périphérique de muscle squelettique et de la glande sous-maxillaire dans la moelle épinière de la souris. C R Acad Sci Paris 290:127–130

Illis LS (1995) Is there a central pattern generator in man? Paraplegia 33:239–240

Ingvar S (1920) Reaction of cells to the galvanic current in tissue cultures. Proc Soc Exp Biol Med 17:198–199

Iwashita Y, Kawaguchi S, Murata M (1994) Restoration of function by replacement of spinal cord segments in the rat. Nature 367:167–170

Jaffe LF (1982) Developmental currents, voltages, and gradients. In: Subtelny S, Green PB (eds) Developmental order: its origin and regulation. Alan R Liss, Inc. New York, pp 183–215

Jaffe LF, Poo M-M (1979) Neurites grow faster toward the cathode than the anode in a steady field. J Exp Zool 209:115–127

Jaffe LF, Nuccitelli R (1974) Electrical controls of development. Annu Rev Biophys Bioeng 6:445–476

Jaffe LF, Robinson KR, Nuccitelli R (1974) Local cation entry and self-electrophoresis as an intracellular localization mechanism. Ann N Y Acad Sci 238:372–389

Jenkins LS, Duerstock BS, Borgens RB (1996) Reduction of the current of injury leaving the amputation inhibits limb regeneration in the red spotted newt. Dev Biol 178:251–262

Kao CC (1974) Comparison of healing processes in transected spinal cords grafted with autogenous brain tissue, sciatic nerve, and nodose ganglion. Exp Neurol 44:424–439

Kao CC, Chang LW (1977) The mechanism of spinal cord cavitation following spinal cord transection. J Neurosurg 46:197–209

Kao CC, Chang LW, Bloodworth JMB (1977) Axonal regeneration across transected mammalian spinal cords: an electron microscopic study of delayed microsurgical nerve grafting. Exp Neurol 54:591–615

Kao CC, Chang LW, Bloodworth JMB (1979) Axonal regeneration across transected spinal cords. Exp Neurol 54:591–615

Kartje GL, Schulz MK, Lopex-Yunez A, Schnell L, Schwab ME (1999) Corticostriatal plasticity is restricted by myelin-associated neurite growth inhibitiors in the adult rat. Ann Neurol 45:778–786

Keirstead SA, Rasminsky M, Fukada T, Carter DA, Aguayo A, Vidal-Sanz M (1989) Electrophysiologic responses in hamster superior colliculus evoked by regenerating retinal axons. Science 246:255–257

Ketchum LD (1982) Peripheral nerve repair. In: Hunt TK (ed) Fundamentals of wound management. Thomas CC, Springfield IL, pp 452–475

Kiehn O, Hounsgaard J, Sillar KT (1997) Basic building blocks of vertebrate spinal central pattern generators. In: Stein PSG, Grillner S, Selverston A, Stuart DG (eds) Neurons, networks, and motor behavior. MIT Press, Cambridge MA, pp 47–59

Kim-Lee MH, Stokes B, Yates A (1992) Reperfusion paradox: a novel mode of glial cell injury. Glia 5:56–64

Kirschner LB (1973) Electrolyte transport across the body surface of freshwater fish and amphibia. In: Ussing HH, Thorn NA, (eds) Transport mechanisms in epithelia. Munksgaard, Copenhagen, pp 447–460

Klusman I, Schwab M (1997) Effects of pro-inflammatory cytokines in experimental spinal cord injury. Brain Res 762:173–184

Knowles JF, Berry M (1978) Effect of enzyme treatment of central nervous system lesions in the rat. Exp Neurol 59:450–454

Krause TL, Fishman HM, Ballinger ML, Bittner GD (1994) Extent and mechanisms of sealing in transected giant axons of squid and earthworms. J Neurosci 14:6638–6651

Krikorian JG, Guth L, Donati EJ (1981) Origin of the connective tissue in the transected rat spinal cord. Exp Neurol 72:698–707

Lance JW (1954) Behavior of pyramidal axons following section. Brain 77:314–324

Lazarov-Speigler O, Soloman ASS, Zeev-Brann AB, Hirschberg DL, Lavie K, Schwartz M (1996) Transplantation of activated macrophages overcomes central nervous system regrowth failure. FASEB 10:1296–1302

Lee J-M, Zipfel GJ, Choi DW (1999) The changing landscape of ischemic brain injury mechanisms. Nature 399:8–14

Lee M-Y, Kim C-J, Sin S-L, Moon S-H, Chun M-H (1998) Increased ciliary neurotrophic factor expression in reactive astrocytes following spinal cord injury in the rat. Neurosci Lett 255:79–82

Le Gros Clark WE (1942) The problem of neuronal regeneration in the central nervous system II: the insertion of peripheral nerve stumps into the brain. J Anat 77:251–259

Leoz O, Arcuate LR (1913) Procesos regenerativos del vervio óptico y retinas con occasión de engertos nerviosos. Trab Lab Invest Boil Univ Madr 11:239–254

Leskovar A, Moriarty LJ, Turek J, Schoenlein IA, Borgens RB (2000) The macrophage in acute neural injury: changes in cell numbers over time and levels of cytokine production in mammalian central and peripheral nervous systems. J Exp Biol 203:1783–1795

Leskovar A, Turek J, Borgens R (2001) Giant multinucleated macrophages occur in acute spinal cord injury. Cell Tissue Res 304:311–315

Letourneau PC, Shattauck TA, Ressler AH (1987) "Push" and "pull" in neurite elongation: observations on the effects of different concentrations of cytochalasin. Cell Motil Cytoskel 8:193–209

Letourneau PC, Kater SB, Macagno ER (1991) The nerve growth cone. Raven Press, New York

Levi-Montalcini R (1987) The nerve growth factor: thirty-five years later. EMBO J 6:1145–1154

Levi-Montalcini R, Angeletti P (1968) Nerve growth factor. Physiol Rev 48:534–569

Li Y, Raisman G (1995) Sprouts from cut corticospinal axons persist in the presence of astrocytic scarring in long-term lesions of the adult rat spinal cord. Exp Neurol 134:102–111

Linliu S, Adey WR, Poo M-M (1984) Migration of cell-surface concanavalin A receptors in pulsed electric fields. J Biophys 45:1211–1217

Liu S, Qu Y, Stewart TJ, Howard MJ, Chakrabortty S, Holekamp TF, McDonald JW (2000) Embryonic stem cells differentiate into oligodendrocytes and myelinate in culture after spinal cord transplantation. Proc Natl Aca Sci U S A 97:6126–6131

Liuzzi FJ, Lasek RJ (1987) Astrocytes block axonal regeneration in mammals by activating the physiological stop pathway. Sci Wash DC 237:642–645

Marder E, Calabrese RL (1996) Principles of rhythmic motor pattern generation. Phys Rev 76:687–717

Marks JD, Pan C-Y, Bushell T, Cromie W, Lee RC (2001) Amphiphilic, tri-block copolymers provide potent, membrane-targeted neuroprotection. FASEB 15:1107–1109

Marsh G, Beams HW (1946) In vitro control of growing chick nerve fibers by applied electric currents. J Cell Comp Physiol 27:139–157

Marsh L, Letourneau PC (1984) Growth of neurites without filopodial or lamellipodial activity in the presence of cytochalasin B. J Cell Biol 99:2041–2047

Martin JP (1967) The basal ganglia and posture. Pittman Med Publishing, London

Maxwell WL (1996) Histopathological changes at central nodes of ranvier after stretch injury. Microsc Res Tech 34:522–535

McCaig CD (1986a) Dynamic aspects of amphibian neurite growth and the effects of an applied electric field. J Physiol 375:55–69

McCaig CD (1986b) Electric fields, contact guidance and the direction of nerve growth. J Embryol Exp Morph 94:245–255

McCaig CD (1989) Nerve growth in the absence of growth cone filopodia and the effects of a small applied electric field. J Cell Sci 93:715–721

McCaig CD, Sangster L, Stewart R (2000) Neurotrophins enchance electric field-directed growth cone guidance and directed nerve branching. Dev Dyn 217:299–308

McCloskey M, Poo M-M (1984) Protein diffusion in cell-membranes some biological implications. Int Rev Cytol 87:19–81

McClosky MA, Liu Z-Y, Poo M-M (1984) Lateral electromigration and diffusion of Fc receptors on rat basophilic leukemia cells: effects of IgE finding. J Cell Biol 99:778–787

McConnell P, Berry M (1982) Regeneration of ganglionic cell axons in the adult mouse retina. Brain Res 241:362–365

McDonald JW, Liu X-Z, Qu Y, Liu S, Mickey SK, Turetsky D, Gottlieb DE, Choi DW (1999) Transplanted embryonic stem cells survive, differentiate and promote recovery in injured rat spinal cord. Nature Med 5(12):1410–1412

McLaughlin S, Poo M-M (1981) The role of electroosmosis in the electric-field-induced movement of charged macromolecules on the surfaces of cells. J Biophys 34:85–93

Menei P, Montero-Menei C, Whittemore SR, Bunge RP, Bunge MB (1998) Schwann cells genetically modified to secrete human BDNF promote enhanced axonal regrowth across transected adult rat spinal cord. Eur J Neurosci 10:607–621

Metcalf MEM, Borgens RB (1994) Weak applied voltages interfere with amphibian morphogenesis and pattern. J Exp Zool 268:322–338

Metcalf MEM, Shi R, Borgens RB (1994) Endogenous ionic currents and voltages in amphibian embryos. J Exp Zool 268:307–322

Ming G-L, Song H-J, Berninger B, Holt CE, Tessier-Lavigne M, Poo M-M (1997) cAMP-dependent growth cone guidance by netrin-1. Neuron 19:1225–1235

Miranda JD, White LA, Marcillo AE, Wilson C, Jagid J, Whittmore S (1999) Induction of Eph B3 after spinal cord injury. Exp Neurol 156:218–222

Mori S, Matsuyama K, Miyashita E, Nakajima K, Asanome M (1995) Basic neurophysiology of primate locomotion. Folia Primatol 66:192–203

Moriarty LJ, Borgens RB (1999) The effect of an applied electrical field on macrophage accumulation within the subactue spinal injury. Rest Neurol Neurosci 14:53–64

Moriarty LJ, Duerstock BS, Bajaj CL, Lin K, Borgens RB (1998) Two- and three-dimensional computer graphic evaluation of the subacute spinal cord injury. J Neurol Sci 155:121–137

Nagata I, Kwana A, Nakatsuju N (1993) Perpendicular contact guidance of CNS neuroblasts on artificial microstructures. Development 117:401–408

Nakahara Y, Gage FH, Tusxynski MH (1996) Grafts of fibroblasts genetically modified to secrete NGF, BDNF, NT-3 or basic FGF elicit differential responses in the adult spinal cord. Cell Transplantation 5:191–204

Napier J (1967) The antiquity of human walking. Sci Am 216:56–66

Nesathurai S (2000) Steroids and spinal cord injury: revisiting the NASCIS 2 and NASCIS 3 trials. J Trauma 48:558–561

Nordlander RH, Singer M (1978) The role of ependyma in regeneration of the spinal cord in the Urodele amphibian tail. J Comp Neurol 180:349–374

Nuccitelli R (1977) Ooplasmic segregation and secretion in the *Pelvetia* egg is accompanied by a membrane-generated electrical current. Dev Biol 62:3–33

Nuccitelli R, Poo M-M, Jaffe LF (1977) Relations between amoeboid movements and electrical currents. J Gen Physiol 69:743–763

O'Callaghan WJ, Speakman T (1963) Axon regeneration in the rat spinal cord. Surg Forum 14:410–411

Ochs S (1977) The early history of nerve regeneration beginning with Crvikshank's observations in 1776. Med Hist 21:261–274

O'Lague PH, Huttner SL (1980) Physiological and morphological studies of rat pheochromocytoma cells (PC12) chemically fused and grown in culture. Proc Natl Acad Sci U S A 77:1701–1705

Oliver JE, Mayhew IG (1983) Neurologic examination and the diagnostic plan. In: Oliver JE Jr, Lorenz MD (eds) Handbook of veterinary neurologic diagnosis. WB Saunders Co, Philadelphia pp 7–13

Orida N, Feldman JD (1982) Directional protrusive pseudopodial activity and motility in macrophages induced by extracellular electric fields. Cell Motil 2:243–255

Orida N, Poo M-M (1978) Electrophorectic movement and localization of acetylcholine receptors in the embryonic muscle cell membrane. Nature 275:31–35

Palmer JS, Cromie WJ, Lee RC (1988) Surfactant administration reduces testicular ischemia-reperfusion injury. J Urology 159:2136–2139

Pasterkamp RJ, DeWinter F, Holtmaat A, Verhaagen J (1998) Evidence for a role of the chemorepellant semaphjorin III and its receptor neuropilin-1 in regeneration of primary olfactory axons. J Neurosci 18:9962–9976

Patel N, Poo M-M (1982) Orientation of neurite growth by extracellular electric fields. J Neurosci 2:483–496

Perry VH, Brown MC (1992) Macrophages and nerve regeneration. Curr Opin Neurobiol 2:679–682

Perry VH, Gordon S (1988) Macrophages and microglia in the nervous system. Trends Neurosci 11:273–277

Perry VH, Gordon S (1991) Macrophages and the nervous system. Int Rev Cytol 125:203–244

Petitjean ME, Pointillart V, Dixmerias F, Wiart L, Sztark F, Lassie P, Thicoipe M, Dabadie P (1998) Traitement médicamenteux de la lésion médullaire traumatique au stade aigu. Ann Fr Anesth Reanim 17:115–122

Pitts LH, Ross AM, Chase GS, Faden AI (1995) Treatment with thyrotropin releasing hormone (TRH) in patients with traumatic spinal cord injuries. J Neurotrauma 12:235–243

Pointillart V, Petitjean ME, Wiart L, Vital JM, Lassie P, Thicoipe M, Dabadie P (2000) Pharmacological therapy of spinal cord injury during the acute phase. Spinal Cord 38:71–76

Poo M-M (1981) In situ electrophoresis of membrane components. Ann Rev Biophys 10:245–276

Poo M-M, Robinson KR (1977) Electrophoresis of concanavalin A receptors along embryonic cell membrane. Nature 265:602–605

Pratt K, Toombs JP, Widmer WR, Borgens RB (1995) Plasma and cerebral spinal fluid concentrations of 4-Aminopyridine following intravenous injection and metered intrathecal delivery in canines. J Neurotrauma 12:23–39

Prewitt CMF, Niesman IR, Kane CJM, Houlé JD (1997) Activated macrophage/microglial cells can promote the regeneration of sensory axons into the injured spinal cord. Experimen Neurol 148:433–443

Raff MC, Whitmore AV, Finn JT (2002) Axonal self-destruction and neurodegeneration. Science 296:868–871

Rajnicek A, Britland S, McCaig C (1997) Contact guidance of CNS neurites on grooved quartz: influence of groove dimensions, neuronal age and cell type. J Cell Sci 110:2905–2913

Rajnicek AM, Robinson KR, McCaig CD (1998) The direction of neurite growth in a weak DC electric field depends on the substratum: contributions of adhesivity and net surface charge. Dev Biol 203:412–423

Rakic P (1971a) Guidance of neurons migrating to the fetal monkey neocortex. Brain Res 33:471–476

Rakic P (1971) Neuron-glia relationship during granule cell migration in developing cerebellar cortex. A Golgi and electromicroscopic study in Macacus rhesus. J Comp Neurol 141:283–312

Ramón y Cajal S (1928) Degeneration and regeneration of the nervous system. Hoffner, New York

Reier PJ, Stensaas LJ, Guth L (1983) The astrocytic scar as an impediment to regeneration in the central nervous system. In: Kao CC, Bunge RP, Reier PJ (eds) Spinal cord reconstruction. Raven Press, New York pp 163–195

Reier PJ, Stokes B, Thompson FJ, Anderson DK (1992) Fetal cell grafts into resection and contusion/compression injuries of the rat and cat spinal cord. Exp Neurol 115:177–188

Reier PJ, Houle JD, Jakeman L, Winialski D, Tessler A (1988) Transplantation of fetal spinal cord tissue into acute and chronic hemisection and contusion lesions of the adult rat spinal cord. Prog Brain Res 78:173–179

Reza JN, Gavazzi I, Cohen J (1999) Neuropilin-1 is expressed on adult mammalian dorsal root ganglion neurons and mediates semaphorin3a/collapsin-1-induced growth cone collapse by small-diameter sensory afferents. Mol Cell Neurosci 14:317–326

Richardson PM, Issa VMK (1984) Peripheral injury enhances central regeneration of primary sensory neurons. Nature 309:791–793

Richardson PM, McGuinness UM, Aguayo AJ (1982) Peripheral nerve autografts to the rat spinal cord: studies with axonal tracing methods. Brain Res 237:147–162

Richardson PM, Issa VMK, Aguayo AJ (1984) Regeneration of long spinal axons in the rat. J Neurocytol 13:165–182

Rivlin AS, Tator CH (1978) Effect of duration of acute spinal cord compression in a new acute cord injury model in the rat. Surg Neurol 10:39–43

Robinson KR (1983) Endogenous electrical current leaves the limb and prelimb region of the Xenopus embryo. Dev Biol 97:203–211

Robinson KR, Jaffe LF (1975) Polarizing fucoid eggs drive a calcium current through themselves. Science 187:70–72

Robinson KR, Cone R (1980) Polarization of fucoid eggs by a calcium ionophore gradient. Science 207:77–78

Robinson KR, Stump RF (1986) Self-generated electrical currents through Xenopus neurulae. J Physiol 352:339–344

Roederer E, Goldberg NH, Cohen MJ (1983) Modification of retrograde degeneration in transected spinal axons of the lamprey by applied DC current. J Neurosci 1:153–160

Rosenberg LJ, Yang DT, Wrathall JR (1999) Effects of the sodium channel blocker tetrodotoxin on acute white matter pathology after experimental contusive spinal cord injury. J Neurosci 19:6122–6133

Ross IB, Tator CH (1991) Further studies of nimodipine in experimental spinal cord injury in the rat. J Neurotrauma 8:229–237

Rovainen CM (1967) Physiological and anatomical studies on large neurons of central nervous system of the sea lamprey. J Neurophysiol 30:1000–1023

Rovainen CM (1974) Synaptic interactions of reticulospinal neurons and nerve cells in the spinal cord of the sea lamprey. J Comp Neur 154:207–224

Sabael BA, Slavin MD, Stein DG (1984) GM-1 ganglion treatment facilitates behavioral recovery from bilateral brain damage. Science Wash DC 255:340–342

Sabael BA, Gottlieb J, Schneider GE (1988) Exogeneous GM 1 gangliosides protect against retrograde degeneration following posterior neocortex lesions in developing hamsters. Brain Res 459:373–380

Sagen J (1997) Transplantation in the spinal cord. In: Lanza R, Langer R, Chick W (eds) Principles of tissue engineering. R G Landes Company, Austin, TX, pp 685–705

Salzman SK, Mendez AA, Sabato S, Lee WA, Ingresoll EB, Choi IH, Fonseca AS, Agresta CA, Freeman GM (1990) Anesthesia influences the outcome from experimental spinal cord injury. Brain Res 521:33–39

Sapolsky RM, Pulsinelli WA (1985) Glucocorticoids potentiate ischemic injury to neurons: therapeutic implications. Science 229:1397–1400

Saveland H, Lijunggren B, Barandt I, Messeter K (1986) Delayed ischemic deterioration in patients with early aneurysm operation and intravenous nimodipine. Neurosurgery 18:146–150

Savio T, Schwab ME (1989) Rats CNS white matter but not gray matter is nonpermissive for neuronal cell adhesion and fiber outgrowth. J Neurosci 9:1126–1133

Schindler R, Mancilla J, Endres S, Ghorbani MR, Vlark SC, Dinarello CA (1990) Correlations and interactions in the production of interleukin 6 (IL-6), IL-1, and tumor necrosis factor (TNF) in human blood mononuclear cells: IL-6 suppresses IL-1 and TNF. Blood 75:40–44

Schlaepfer WW (1974) Calcium-induced degeneration of axoplasm in isolated segments of rat peripheral nerve. Brain Research 69:203–215

Schnell L, Schwab M (1990) Axonal regeneration in the rat spinal cord produced by an antibody against myelin-associated neurite growth inhibitors. Nature 343:269–272

152

Schnell L, Schneider R, Kolbeck R, Barde Y-A, Schwab M (1994) Neurotropin-3 enhances sprouting of corticospinal tract during development and after adult spinal cord lesion. Nature 367:170–173

Schnell L, Fearn S, Schwab M, Perry V, Anthoney DC (1999) Cytokine-induced acute inflammation in the brain and spinal cord. J Neuropath Exp Neurol 58:245–254

Schwab ME, Bartholdi D (1996) Degeneration and regeneration of axons in the lesioned spinal cord. Physiol Rev 76:319–370

Schwab M, Kapfhammer J, Bandtlow CE (1993) Inhibitors of neurite growth. Ann Rev Neurosci 16:565–595

Shi R, Borgens RB (1994) Embryonic neuroepithelium sodium transport, the resulting physiological potential, and cranial development. Dev Biol 165:105–116

Shi R, Borgens RB (1995) Three-dimensional gradients of voltage during development of the nervous system as invisible coordinates for the establishment of the embryonic pattern. Dev Dyn 202:101–114

Shi R, Borgens RB (1999) Acute repair of crushed guinea pig spinal cord by polyethylene glycol. J Neurophysiol 81:2406–2414

Shi R, Borgens RB (2000) Anatomical repair of nerve membranes in crushed mammalian spinal cord with polyethylene glycol. J Neurocytol 29:633–643

Shi R, Borgens RB, Blight AR (1999) Functional reconnection of severed mammalian spinal cord axons with polyethylene glycol. J Neurotrauma 16:727–738

Shi R, Pryor JD (2000) Temperature dependence of membrane sealing following transection in mammalian spinal cord axons. Neuroscience 98:157–166

Shi R, Asano T, Wining NC, Blight AR (2000) Control of membrane sealing in injured mammalian spinal cord axons. J Neurophysiol 84:1763–1769

Shimizu I, Oppenheim RW, O'Brien M, Shneiderman A (1990) Anatomical and functional recovery following spinal cord transection in the chick embryo. J Neurobiol 21:918–937

Short DJ, El Masry WS, Jones PW (2000) High-dose methylprednisolone in the management of acute spinal cord injury – a systematic review from a clinical perspective. Spinal Cord 38:273–286

Simpson SB (1968) Morphology of the regenerated spinal cord in the lizard Anolis Carolinensis. J Comp Neurol 134:193–210

Singer M (1954) Induction of regeneration of the forelimb of the post-metamorphic frog by augmentation of the nerve supply. J Exp Zool 126:419–471

Singer M, Norlander RH, Eger M (1979) Axonal guidance during embryogenesis and regeneration in the spinal cord of the newt: the blueprint hypothesis of neuronal pathway patterning. J Comp Neurol 185:1–22

Sisken BF, Smith SD (1975) The effect of minute directed electrical currents on cultured chick trigeminal ganglia. J Embryol Morphol 33:29–41

Smith AG (2001) Embryo-derived stem cells: of mice and men. Annu Rev Cell Dev Biol 17:435–462

Snow DM, Letourneau PC (1992) Neurite outgrowth on a step gradient of chondroitin sulfate proteoglycan (CS-PG). J Neurobiol 23:322–336

Snow DM, Lemmon V, Carrino DA, Caplan AI, Silver J (1990) Sulfated proteoglycans in astroglial barriers inhibit neurite outgrowth in vitro. Exp Neurol 190:111–130

Snow DM, Watanabe M, Letourneau PC, Silver J (1991) A chondroitin sulfate proteoglycan may influence the direction of retinal ganglion cell outgrowth. Development 113:1473–1485

Snow DM, Atkinson PB, Hassinger TD, Letourneau PC, Kater SB (1994) Chondroitin sulphate proteoglycan elevates cytoplasmic calcium in DRG neurons. Dev Biol 166:87–100

Snow DM, Brown EM, Letourneau PC (1996) Growth cone behavior in the presence of soluble chondroitin sulfate proteoglycan (CSPG), compared to behavior on CSPG bound to laminin or fibronectin. Int J Dev Neurosci 14:331–349

Somerson SK, Stokes BT (1987) Functional analysis of an electromechanical spinal cord injury device. Exp Neurol 96:82–96

Song HJ, Poo M-M (1999) Signal transduction underlying growth cone guidance by diffusible factors. Curr Opin Neurobiol 9:355–363

Song HJ, Ming GL, Poo M-M (1997) cAMP-induced switching inturning direction of nerve growth cones. Nature 388:275–279

Stewart R, Erskine L, McCaig CD (1995) Calcium channel subtypes and intracellular calcium stores modulate electric field-stimulated and oriented nerve growth. Dev Biol 171:340–351

Stollberg J, Fraser SE (1988) Acetylcholine receptors and concanavilin A-binding sites on cultured Xenopus muscles: electrophoresis, diffusion and aggregation. J Cell Biol 106:1723–1734

Strautman AF, Cook RJ, Robinson KR (1990) The distribtion of free calcium in transected spinal axons and it modulation by applied electrical fields. J Neurosci 10:3564–3575

Stys PK (1998) Anoxic and ischemic injury of myelinated axons in CNS white matter: from mechanistic concepts to therapeutics. J Cereb Blood Flow Metab 18:2–25

Stys PK, Waxman SG, Ransom BR (1991) Reverse operation of the Na$^+$–Ca^{2+} exchanger mediates Ca^{2+} influx during anoxia in mammalian CNS white matter. Ann N Y Acad Sci 639:328–332

Stys PK, Waxman SG, Ransom BR (1992) Ionic mechanisms of anoxic injury in mammalian CNS white matter: role of Na$^+$ channels and Na$^+$–Ca^{2+} exchanger. J Neurosci 12:430–439

Stys PK, Sontheimer H, Ransom BR, Waxman SG (1993) Noninactivating, tetrodotoxin-sensitive Na$^+$ conductance in rat optic nerve axons. Proc Natl Acad Sci U S A 90:6976–6980

Sugar O, Gerard RW (1940) Spinal cord regeneration in the rat. J Neurophysiol 3:1–19

Tardieu C, Aurengo A, Tardieu B (1993) New method of three-dimensional anaylsis of bipedal locomotion for the study of displacements of the body and body-parts centers of mass in man and non-human primates: evolutionary framework. Am J Phys Anthropol 90:455–476

Tarlov IM (1957) Spinal cord compression: mechanisms of paralysis and treatment. Charles C. Thomas, Springfield, IL, pp 1–147

Tator C (1995) Clinical manifestations of acute spinal cord injury. In: Benxel EC, Tator CH (eds) Contemporary management of spinal cord injury. American Association of Neurological Surgeons, Park Ridge, IL, pp 15–26

Tator CH, Fehlings MG (1991) Review of the secondary injury theory of acute spinal cord trauma with emphasis on vascular mechanisms. J Neurosurg 75:15–26

Tator CH, Deecke L (1972) Normothermic vs hypothermic perfusion in treatment of acute experimental spinal cord injury. Surgical Forum 23:435–438

Theodore N, Sonntag VKH (2000) Spinal surgery: The past century and the next. Neurosurgery 46:767–777

Theriault A, Diamond J (1988a) Nociceptive cutaneous stimuli evoke localized contractions in a skeletal muscle. J Neurophysiol 60:446–462

Theriault A, Diamond J (1988b) Intrinsic organization of the rat cutaneus trunci motor nucleus. J Neurophysiol 60:463–477

Thomas PK (1988) Clinical aspects of PNS regeneration. In: Waxman SG (ed) Advances in neurology: functional recovery in neurological disease. (vol 47) Raven Press, New York

Toffano S, Savoini G, Maroni F, Lombarcalza MG, Agnati LF (1983) GM-1 ganglioside stimulates the reaction of dopaminergic neurons in the central nervous system. Res 261:163–166

Toombs JP, Bauer MS (1993) Intervertebral disc disease. In: Slatter D (ed) Textbook of small animal surgery. W B Saunders Company, pp 1070–1087

Treherne JM, Woodward SKA, Varga ZM, Ritchie JM, Nicholls JG (1992) Restoration of conduction and growth of axons through injured spinal cord of neonatal opossum in culture. Proc Natl Acad Sci U S A 89:431–434

Trump BF, Balentine JD, Berezesky IK (1998) Mechanisms of cellular injury and death. J Neurotrauma 5:215–218

Tuszynski MH, Murai Blesch A, Grill R, Miller I (1997) Functional characterization of NGF-secreting cell grafts to the acutely injured spinal cord. Cell Transplantation 6:361–368

Tuszynski MH, Gabriel K, Gerhardt K, Szollar S (1999) Human spinal cord retains substantial structural mass in chronic stages after injury. J Neurotrauma 16:523–531

Vacanti MP, Leonard JL, Dore B, Bonassar LJ, Cao Y, Stachelek SJ, Vacanti JP, O'Connell F, Yu CS, Farwell AP, Vacanti CA (2001) Tissue-engineered spinal cord. Transplant Proc 33:592–598

Vanable JW Jr (1989) Integumentary potentials and wound healing. In: Borgens RB, Robinson KR, Vanable JW Jr, McGinnis ME (eds) Electric fields in vertebrate repair. Alan R Liss, Inc, New York, pp 171–214

Vescovi A, Snyder EY (1999) Establishment and properties of neural stem cell clones: plasticity in vitro and in vivo. Brain Pathol 9:569–598

Vidal-Sanz M, Bray G, Villegas-Perez M, Thanos S, Aguayo A (1987) Axonal regeneration and synapse formation in the superior colliculus by retinal ganglion cells in the adult rat. J Neurosci 7:2894–2902

Vikhanski L (2001) In search of the lost cord: solving the mystery of spinal cord regeneration. Joseph Henry Press, Washington DC

Wallace MC, Tator CH, Young W (1987) Recovery of spinal cord function induced by direct current stimulation of the injured rat spinal cord. Neurosurgery 20:878–884

Warner AE (1985) Factors controlling the early development of the nervous system. In: Edelman GM, Gall WE, Cowan WM (eds) Molecular bases of neural development. John Wiley and Sons, NewYork, pp 11–34

Weiss P (1934) In vitro experiments on the factors determining the course of the outgoing nerve fibre. J Exp Zool 68:393–448

Wenk CA, Thallmair M, Kartje GL, Schwab ME (1999) Increased corticofugal plasticity after unilateral cortical lesions combined with neutralization of the IN-1 antigen in adult rats. J Comp Neurol 410:143–157

White RJ, Yashon D, Albin MS (1969) The technique of localized spinal cord hypothermia in the human. Proc V A Spinal Cord Injury Conf, pp 58–60

Wickelgren I (1998) Teaching the spinal cord to walk. Science 279:319–321

Wictorin K, Lagenaur CF, Lund RD, Björklund A (1991) Efferent projections to the host brain from intrastriatal striatal mouse-to-rat grafts: time course and tissue-type specificity as revealed by a mouse-specific neuronal marker. Eur J Neurosci 3:86–101

Windle WF (1956) Regeneration of axons in the vertebrate central nervous system. Physl Rev 36:427–440

Windle WF, Chambers WW (1950) Regeneration in the spinal cord of the cat and dog. J Comp Neurol 93:241–257

Wojcik M, Vlas J Oerelt-Nowak B (1982) The stimulating effect of ganglioside injections on the recovery of choline acetyltransferase and acetylcholinesterase activities in the hippocampus of the rat after septal lesions. Neuroscience 7:495–499

Wood MR, Cohen JJ (1979) Synaptic regeneration in identified neurons of the lamprey spinal cord. Science 206:344

Wolfe DL, Hayes KC, Hsieh JT, Potter PJ (2001) Effects of 4-aminopyridine on motor-evoked potentials in patients with spinal cord injury: a double-blinded, placebo-controlled crossover trial. J Neurotrauma 18:757–771

Wrathall JR, Choiniere D, Teng YD (1994) Dose-dependent reduction of tissue loss and functional impairment after spinal cord trauma with the AMPA/kainite antagonist NBQX. J Neurosci 14:6598–6607

Yakovleva LA (1954) Der ersatz eines defects im Rückenmark durch homotransplants des degenerierten nervus ischiadicus (in Russian) Dolk Akad Navk SSSR N S 98:104–1043

Yoganandan A, Halliday, Dickman C, Benxel E (1999) Practical anatomy and fundamental biomechanics in spine surgery. (vol 1) In: Benzel E (ed) Churchill Livingston, New York, pp 93–118

Young W (1993) Secondary injury mechanisms in acute spinal cord injury. J Emerg Med 11:13–22

Young SH, Poo M-M (1983) Topographical rearrangement of acetylcholine-receptors alters channel kinetics. Nature 304:161–163

Zelena J (1969) Bidirectional shift of mitochondria in axons after injury. In: Barondes S (ed) Cellular dynamics of the neuron. Symp Int Soc Cell Biol 8:73–94

Zelena J, Lubinska L, Gutman E (1968) Accumulation of organelles at the ends of interrupted axons. Z Zellforsch Mikrosk Anat 91:200–219

Z'Graggen WJ, Metz GAS, Kartje GL, Thallmair M, Schwab ME (1998) Functional recovery and enhanced corticofugal plasticity after unilateral pyramidal tract lesion and blockade of myelin-associated neurite growth inhibitors in adult rats. J Neurosci 18:4744–4757

Zheng JQ, Felder M, Connor JA, Poo M (1994) Turning of nerve growth cones induced by neurotransmitters. Nature 368:140–144

Zheng JQ, Wan JJ and Poo M-M (1996) Essential role of filopodia in chemotropic turning of nerve growth cone induced by a glutamate gradient. J Neurosci 16:1140–1149

Subject Index

oscillating field stimulation   27, 107
oxygen deprivation   16

P
panniculus reflex   36
paraplegia   7
paraplegic dog   52
parenchyma   8
paresis   7
patellar   115
PEG nontoxic   130
peripheral nerve bridge   44, 56
phagocytic cell   102
Plastek C   86
– M   86
poloxamer 188   135
poloxamine 1107   135
Poly-L-lysine   86
polyethylene glycol (PEG)   119
polymer   119
– injection   129
polymeric tube   44
polypropylene oxide   135
postural control   29
potential difference   71
primitive streak in the chick embryo   68
progressive myonecrosis   135
propriospinal fiber   29
proteoglycans   47
pseudoembryo   78
Pyromen   25, 102

Q
quadriplegia   7

R
radial glial cell   78
Rakic, Pasco   47, 78
Ramón y Cajal, Santiago   13
raphe nucleus   106
reactive astrocyte   21
– reinnervation   42
reconnection of proximal and distal segments
  of spinal cord   121
recording chamber   119
red nucleus   106
reflex   8
– circuit   30
Reier, Paul   59
repair   54
reperfusion injury   16
resistivity   67
respiration   12
restoration   51
reticulospinal neurons   91
retrograde degeneration   43, 95

– labeling   101
– transport   39
rhizoid   68
– of the fucus egg   68
right lateral hemisection   105
rTAPA (target of the antiproliferative
  antibody)   22

S
salt bridges   91
scar barrier hypothesis   19
– plug   101
Schlaepfer, William   15
Schwab, Martin   62
Schwann cell   11
sciatic   115
sealing   123
secondary axotomy   119
short circuit K^+ current   52
silica   23
Singer, Marcus   47
Silver, Jerry   21
skin battery   70
– wound   68
somatosensory evoked potential (SSEP)   116
– testing   111, 115
spinal roots   7
– shock   8, 34
– stepping   31
spinothalamic   4
– tract   3
standard of care   1
Stanley Cohen   49
stem cell   60
stepping and gait   31
stretch-activated potassium channel   49
subacute   17
subcutaneous injection   129
superficial pain   113, 115
superoxide anion   16
supraspinal control   29
surfactant   119
syncytium   71
systemic Ca^{++} channel blockade   54

T
tantalum marker   96
tenascin   47
tetraplegia   7
tetrodotoxin   55
TGF-β 50
thallus   68
thyroid-releasing hormone   27
tibialis   115
TNF-3   23
transection   9